Nu

MW01295440

Understanding The Basics:

Nutrition 101, Healthy Eating, And Weight Loss

Lose Weight And Feel Great!

3rd Edition

By

Nicholas Bjorn

Nicholas Bjorn

© Copyright 2014 - All rights reserved.

professional advice.

Table of Contents

Nicholas Bjorn

Introduction

I want to thank you and congratulate you for purchasing, **"Nutrition: Understanding The Basics: Nutrition 101, Healthy Eating. And Weight Loss – Lose Weight And Feel Great!"**

This book contains proven steps and strategies on how to lose weight and keep it off. You will learn what the basics of nutrition are all about and what you need to do to ensure that you are in peak health at all times. You can definitely lose weight naturally and quickly by eating what's right for you!

With the help of this book, you will learn the importance of reading food labels and making sure that you get the right amount of nutrients during each meal. This will ensure that you not only lose weight, but also keep the weight off while preventing disease, thus leading to a happier, healthier life. Lose weight and feel great the right way!

Thanks again for purchasing this book, and I hope you enjoy it!

Nicholas Bjorn

Chapter 1: The Basics Of Nutrition

With the rise in obesity levels in most of the Western world and with its increasing prevalence across many under-developed countries, there have been hundreds of diets that have been promoted both to reduce weight and to maintain a healthy lifestyle. The problem is that whilst most of them are great and offer impressive results initially, their long-term effects may not be so beneficial. Whether we want to reduce weight or simply eat a healthier diet. the solution does not lie in the latest fad eating regime. Instead, what we need is a system of eating that is both healthy and sustainable over the long term.

Well, the solution to that problem may not be as complicated as we may think. Many modern health problems, or the lack thereof, stem from changes in eating habits made over the last fifty years. Prior to World War II, the average male in London consumed over three thousand calories per day, and yet, obesity was not the problem that it now is. Sure, there was, by necessity, more exercise being done, but jogging and aerobics were not around then. Exercise tended to be moderate and performed within the course of general daily routine, such as riding or walking to work or using a push mower rather than a drive-on one. If that is the case, what changes have been made to our modern lifestyles that facilitate the increase in weight in such a large proportion of our societies?

To enable ease of access to a healthy diet, the government developed a system known as the food plate. We will start by taking a broad look at this system, and from there, we will look at some easy ways to change eating habits for the better into more detail. These habits are not only healthier but, in many cases, they are cheaper, too. The fact is that much of the obesity explosion we have been witnessing has taken place in the poorer communities of our society. and any changes made need to be accessible to both rich and poor alike.

If you want to live a healthy and well-balanced life, it is important that you maintain a well-balanced diet. The problem is, not all people know how to make sure that their meals are balanced and that they are eating the right kinds of foods to get all the nutrients that their bodies need. It is also important to know how much of these foods you should be eating.

In 2011, the Food Plate replaced the Food Pyramid as an easier means of showing people what they should eat for every meal. It's a way of zoning your plate and making sure that you fill your plate up with the right food choices. This Food Plate is known as "MyPlate" and is the current nutritional guide published by the United States Department of Agriculture.

Basically, a food plate should consist of at least 75% vegetables, and then the remaining 25% should be partitioned between protein, grains, and fruits. A small saucer of dairy can also be included. The notes below will help you understand the partitions of the Food Plate better:

Vegetables

In the early nineties, the World Health Organization came up with the five-a-day fruit and veg plan that most people are familiar with. A significant amount of servings have been added since then, and most health organizations now recommend between seven and thirteen cups of fruits or vegetables per day, with vegetables making up the majority. The problem is that even on the five-a-day system, only thirty percent of the population achieved the WHO target. The importance of vegetables in a diet cannot be overstressed. Vegetables are four times healthier than fruit, and with the exception of those high in starch, they can be eaten without limit and are thus great and healthy snacks to grab when you are feeling hungry.

Many of the dark green vegetables are known as superfoods, including spinach, kale, broccoli, and Brussel sprouts. These superfoods have a lot of benefits that many people don't know about. The biggest benefit with these foods is the high amount of nutrients that is present in them. These foods are more nutrient dense than any other vegetables on the list. Spinach is especially good, with plenty of vitamin K, which helps promote bone health, lots of antioxidants, and plenty of anti-inflammatories. It's no wonder spinach is often considered one of the best superfoods.

Many of the red and orange vegetables have plenty of nutrients which not only promote bone health, but eye health as well. Nutrients like zeaxanthin plays an important role in the health of your eyes. They help protect your eyes when they are exposed to UV rays and other harmful high-energy light. Lycopene is another antioxidant that is incredibly beneficial to your body. With this antioxidant, it can protect your body from any harm that pesticides can induce on your body. Pesticides are full of harmful chemicals that people digest on a daily basis. Lycopene is a great way to help stop any damage in its tracks.

Starchy vegetables are a great source of fiber. Fiber is one of those nutrients some people don't consume enough of. This aids in digestion and helps keep your blood sugar levels stable, making fiber an incredibly important nutrient. B-vitamins are also prominent in starchy vegetables. Many scientists agree that these vitamins can reduce the risk of heart attack and stroke. They also aid in promoting positive moods. They interact with the dopamine and serotonin levels in the brain and guarding against memory loss. Most adults do not eat the recommended amount of starchy vegetables that they should. One cup of potatoes can go a long way.

There are tons of benefits with beans and peas. Many beans are a significant source of protein, which is beneficial to those who are vegetarian or vegan. They are also full of different minerals, including copper, iron, magnesium, and phosphorus. Copper is very important throughout life, but infants who are deprived of copper by being given cow's milk may have many issues as they get older. Copper is stored in the liver. A deficiency can lead to osteoporosis, increased risk of infection, impaired neurological growth, and stunted growth. Adults and adolescents don't need a significant amount of copper, only 900 micrograms a day.

Peas, on the other hand, have some different benefits. While many of the nutrients are similar, the top two nutrients in green peas specifically are vitamin K and manganese. Vitamin K is important in bone health and also plays a huge role in making sure your blood clots correctly. Manganese also has a ton of benefits for your bones. It's also used as a co-enzyme in the metabolism, helping with digestion.

People who eat large quantities of vegetables have a significantly lower risk of premature death than those who do not. Those with a high intake are also much less likely to get cancer. Adults should eat at least 2 ½ to 3 cups of vegetables each day. It's suggested to eat different kinds of vegetables in various colors. This variety will you remain enthusiastic in consuming your food, aside from offering a wider range of nutrients. Below is a chart that would enable you to become familiar with the various types of vegetables:

Dark Green Vegetables	Romaine Lettuce, Spinach, Collard Greens, Bok Choy, Broccoli, Spinach, Kale, Dark Green Leafy Lettuce, Mustard Greens, Turnip Greens
Red and Orange Vegetables	Butternut Squash, Acorn Squash, Carrots, Red Peppers, Orange Peppers, Pumpkin, Hubbard Squash, Tomatoes, Sweet Potatoes
Starchy Vegetables	Corn, Cassava, Green Bananas, Cow peas, Green Peas, Potatoes, Green Lima Beans, Taro, Water Chestnuts, Plantains
Beans and Peas	Garbanzos, Black-Eyed Peas, Black Beans, Lentils, Kidney Beans, Pinto Beans, Navy Beans, Split Peas, Soy Beans, White Beans
Other Vegetables	Artichokes, Asparagus, Cauliflower, Cabbage, Beets, Bean Sprouts, Cucumbers, Celery, Eggplant, Green Peppers, Green Beans, Onions, Okra, Mushrooms, Iceberg Lettuce, Zucchini, Wax Beans, Turnips

Protein

The average male should eat at least fifty-six grams of protein per day, whilst the average female should eat forty-six grams daily. These figures are for the average sedentary adult, and many active people should be eating more. Protein is what our bodies use to manufacture things. In short, our bodies are like small, highly advanced factories that are constantly rebuilding and repairing themselves. They are forever building muscle, growing hair and nails, repairing organs, and strengthening bones. The main building block for all these activities comes from protein, and that is also the reason why it is quite tricky to determine the exact daily intake needed. This amount will vary according to how much exercise we do, what age we are, what our body mass is, etc. Without protein, it would be impossible to maintain life as we know it. Protein is also highly sating to the appetite and can therefore be a useful tool in controlling calorie intake.

Most protein comes in the form of animal products, particularly red meat. If your choice is not to eat red meat, then you can eat seafood in place of meat to make sure you are including enough protein in your meals.

If you want the most protein in your meat, pork tenderloin, chicken, turkey, and steak have the most protein per bite. These are great for people who are working out often and want to build up muscle. Lean meat is definitely the best when it comes to this, as there is less fat. You'll be able to eat the meat without worrying about putting on too much weight.

Chicken is the most widely eaten kind of poultry in the world, and for good reason. There is a lot of protein while also being beneficial in other ways. This has an amino acid called tryptophan, which gives you something of a comforting feeling. This helps bring your serotonin levels up, making you feel happier. Chicken is rich in phosphorus, which promotes teeth and bone health. It also helps make sure that your kidneys, liver, and central nervous system function regularly. If you want a boost in your metabolism, chicken would be a good food to eat. Niacin is a B-vitamin that can help guard against cancer and other types of DNA damaging diseases.

Seafood is a great alternative to other meats. Not only do they have plenty of protein, but they have a ton of vitamins and minerals, some of which are harder to find in certain foods. Fish oil, for example, has a multitude of benefits. It has omega-3s, which decreases the symptoms of depression, hypertension, ADHD, joint pain, arthritis, and some chronic skin ailments. It also helps with weight loss, fertility, pregnancy, and increasing energy. Eating some fish every week will help reduce your chances for a heart attack by nearly half.

Eggs are a great source of protein. The protein is focused in the whites of the eggs. Some people prefer to eat only the eggs whites because of the protein that's in them. Plus, they have plenty of other nutrients, including vitamin B-2, selenium, vitamin D, zinc, iron, and copper. Selenium is important in keeping your immune system healthy. With weight loss, eggs can be an incredibly good for helping to keep you feeling full for a lot longer, as well as giving you energy. Biotin is the big thing in helping with metabolizing fat. This can be a hard thing for your body to do, so it's good that there is something that can help with fat metabolism.

Nuts and seeds are another protein filled food. This can be added to your meals in many different ways, including on salads, in cereals, or just as a snack food. These are also filled with healthy mono and polyunsaturated fats, which are helpful for managing inflammation and the normal structure of your body. Fiber is also a big part of nuts and seeds. This is a great nutrient which helps keep your body feeling fuller for a lot longer, making these a great snack food.

Beans and peas are some of the foods with protein and one of the best sources of protein for vegans and vegetarians. Most of the benefits for these foods are mentioned up above in the vegetable section.

Processed soy products also are a good source of protein. Along with that, they also have plenty of vitamins and minerals, like B-vitamins and iron. These are great for vegans and vegetarians. The benefits of tofu include having eight essential amino acids available in this. It has been shown to reduce the possibility of having prostate and breast cancer, cardiovascular disease, osteoporosis, type-2 diabetes, age-related brain diseases, or liver damage. Some scientists have seen that people who eat too many soy products can have issues later in life because of isoflavones. These can lead to estrogen overload in both men and women and can cause a lot of problems later in life.

For those who choose not to eat meat at all, there are some plants that are fairly high in protein as well. Examples of foods that are rich in protein include the following:

Meat	Ham, Lamb, Beef, Veal, Pork, Bison, Venison, Giblets, Liver
Poultry	Duck, Chicken, Turkey, Goose, Ground Turkey/ Chicken
Seafood	Cod, Catfish, Haddock, Flounder, Herring, Halibut, Pollock, Mackerel,

	Salmon, Porgy, Sea Bass, Salmon, Swordfish, Snapper, Tuna, Trout, Clams. Crayfish, Crab, Scallops. Oysters, Mussels, Lobsters, Shrimp, Octopus, Anchovies, Sardines
Eggs	Chicken Eggs, Quale Eggs
Nuts and Seeds	Cashews, Almonds, Mixed Nuts, Hazelnuts, Peanuts, Pistachios, Pecans, Sesame Seeds, Pumpkin Seeds, Walnuts, Sunflower Seeds
Beans and Peas	Black Beans, Bean Burgers, Chick Peas, Black Eyed Peas, Soy Beans, Split Beans, Pinto Beans, Navy Beans, Lentils, Lima Beans
Processed Soy Products	Veggie Burgers, Tofu, Texturized Vegetable Protein, Tempeh

Grains

It's also important for adults to eat at least 5 to 7 ounces of grains each day. It would be best to eat whole grains, as they contain the highest amount of nutrients.

Whole grains have tons of benefits, including having a reduced risk of stroke, heart attack, and type 2 diabetes. There are tons of nutrients in whole grains, all of which aid in keeping these things at bay. Iron is important in the red blood cells and preventing anemia. Anemia can cause fatigue and reduce your energy by a lot, so making sure you have a proper amount of iron in your diet is crucial. Whole wheat pasta is a great source of fiber, which promotes digestive health and reduces the chances of type 2 diabetes.

Refined grains do lose some of the benefits that whole grains have and don't contain any fiber. However, they do have certain B-vitamins and iron, which are put back into the grains after they are refined. As long as the average adult still gets a good amount of fiber in their diet, having some refined grains is not the end of the world.

Pastas are a great source of carbohydrates. These carbs will give you energy for a while, helping you stay energized for a longer period of time. Selenium is present in all types of pasta, which is a mineral that activates antioxidant enzymes, preventing molecular damage in your cells. Folate is very prominent in pasta as well, with about 42 percent of the daily folate intake in a serving of pasta.

Breakfast cereals have tons of vitamins and minerals, but the amount changes depending on the type of breakfast cereal. Many cereals are rich in fiber, including oatmeal and bran cereals. Corn flakes are rich in thiamine, which helps immensely with carbohydrate metabolism and energy production. While they might not be as high in fiber as some of the other cereals, they are high in iron. This is important to not only maintain healthy blood levels, but also to keep the brain alert.

These include brown rice, pasta, oatmeal, and whole wheat cereal. Here's a grain chart for you with additional options:

| **Whole Grains** | Brown Rice, Amaranth, Millet, Bulgur, Buckwheat, Triticale, Popcorn, Oatmeal, Quinoa, Whole Grain Cornmeal, Whole Grain Barley, Whole Wheat Pasta, |

	Whole Wheat Crackers, Whole Wheat Rolls and Sandwich Buns, Wild Rice
Refined Grains	Corn Tortillas, Cornbread, Crackers, Couscous, Grits, Flour Tortillas, Pitas, Noodles, White Bread, Pretzels, White Rice, White Sandwich Buns and Rolls
Pastas	Macaroni, Spaghetti
Breakfast Cereals	Muesli, Whole Wheat Cereal Flakes, Corn Flakes

Fruits

Fruits are always delicious and are great to eat as a snack or dessert. Adults should try to eat around 1 ½ to 2 cups of fruit each day, be it raw fruit or fruit juice.

When it comes to fruits, some people think the daily consumption should be high. However, many people forget that there are natural sugars in these fruits. Vegetables should be more frequently eaten than fruits, but that doesn't mean fruits should be forgotten. Everyone has heard the saying 'An apple a day keeps the doctor away' and it's common knowledge that it isn't entirely an old wives' tale. Apples are full of antioxidants, which help with fighting off diseases and preventing future diseases. They are one of the best fruits to eat, since they do so many different things to help with your body.

Berries are a little different. They are most well-known for their phytochemicals, which help by preventing damage to the cells. The great thing about this is berries can be eaten by the handful. Other fruits are generally eaten one at a time rather than in bunches, making berries a great snack food. This can also be a great food to help lower your cholesterol. Strawberries, red raspberries, and bilberries are the best berries for heart health.

Melons are another fruit, one which has some surprising benefits. They have little to no fat or saturated fat and have a lot of vitamins and minerals. Vitamin C and A are the biggest vitamins in these melons. Vitamin C is very important in giving you the essentials that you need for maintaining your tissues and healing injuries. Vitamin A is important in keeping up your immune system, keeping your teeth healthy, and helping your vision. Plus, melons have some weight loss benefits, since they are a sweet, sugary dessert that isn't at the same unhealthy level that other sugary sweets are.

Fruit juice isn't the first choice when it comes to getting your recommended fruit intake. This tends to have more sugars and things that you shouldn't be drinking. However, 100% fruit juice is a much better choice. This can be freshly squeezed, which is the best idea when it comes to drinking juice, as it comes directly from the fruits. Though juice is a good idea, try to limit how much of it you drink. You don't want to consume too much sugar.

Take a look at this fruit chart for more options:

Commonly Eaten Fruits	Apricots, Apples, Kiwis, Cherries, Bananas, Grapes, Nectarines, Mangoes, Limes, Lemon, Plums, Pineapples, Papaya, Pears, Tangerines, Raisins, Prunes, Oranges, Peaches
Berries	Raspberries, Strawberries, Blueberries

Melons	Honeydew, Cantaloupe, Watermelon
100% Fruit Juice	Grape, Apple, Orange, Grapefruit

Dairy

Three servings of dairy should be consumed daily. It would be best to choose fat-free or low-fat dairy to ensure that weight loss is achieved more effectively.

Everyone knows that milk is a good source of calcium. Calcium, of course, helps with keeping bones strong and healthy. Right along with that, vitamin D is an important vitamin in keeping good levels of calcium and phosphorus. This is found in milk, so you don't have to worry about not having enough.

There are many different kinds of cheese, all of which have different kinds of fat content. Some cheeses, like goat cheese, feta cheese, and blue cheese have a higher fat content than others do. These cheeses have been given a lot of 'fillers' which add to their flavor, but make them much more concentrated in fat. Other cheeses, like part-skim mozzarella, parmesan, or grated Romano are generally lower in fat. There are also low-fat and fat-free versions of different cheeses that are available to buy. Outside of the fat content, you'll be getting plenty of vitamins and nutrients in any cheese.

Yogurt is rapidly becoming a very popular option as a snack food or breakfast food. Any grocery store will be overrun with yogurt options in the dairy section. Yogurt, since it is made from milk, has all of the benefits of milk, including calcium, potassium, vitamin B-2, and vitamin B-12. Probiotics are another part of yogurt, one which some people are skeptical about. These are good bacteria that is found in your digestive system. It helps fight off infections by boosting the immune system. Yogurt also has a part in reducing the chances of osteoporosis, since both calcium and vitamin D are in yogurt. These two nutrients have been linked to keeping bones healthy and strong.

Here are further examples of dairy sources:

Milk	Low-Fat, Skim, Reduced Fat, Whole Milk, Lactose-Reduced, Lactose-Free, Flavored Milk (Strawberry, Chocolate)
Cheese	Mozzarella, Cheddar, Swiss, Parmesan, Cottage Cheese, Ricotta, American
Yogurt	Low Fat, Fat Free, Whole Milk Yogurt, Reduced Fat
Soy	Soy Milk, Soy Beverages
Milk-Based Desserts	Ice Milk, Pudding, Ice Cream, Frozen Yogurt

Chapter 2: Dietary Guidelines

Control Calorie Intake

As a rule of thumb, if you control your calorie intake and burn the same amount of calories as you consume, your weight will be maintained at the same level. Whilst this generally makes good sense, there are several problems that we may quickly encounter here. In the first place, counting calories accurately can be complicated. It has been proven in several broad-scale studies that people counting their calorie intake are notoriously bad at getting the figures right. We almost always tend to underestimate the calories we consume and overestimate the amount we burn. Moreover, not all calories are created equal.

Some people will be able to develop a regime of balancing their exercise levels against their calorie intake and then either lose weight or maintain the weight they are targeting. It is definitely a good idea to have knowledge of calorific values so that we can keep a rough idea of where we stand in terms of the amount of food we eat. However, it is just as important to reach a point in which we are eating a healthy diet that provides our daily energy needs without having to run through a convoluted calculation as to how much a particular food item weighs and how many calories it is going to provide.

It would be simpler to ensure that you are eating a healthy, well-cooked diet of fresh vitamin-packed food rather than having to start with some grand calculation. Most people our grandparent's age had no idea what their calorie intake was or even what it should be on a daily basis. Do you know, for example, how many calories you will burn in the course of a normal workday or how much that figure would change if you were to jog for an hour? Hopefully, by the time you finish this book, you will have a clearer idea, but I am still not promoting constant calorie calculation, even with the help of modern calorie counting apps and calorie counting books that are currently available. Instead, I hope that by the time you have finished this book, you can look at an apple or vegetable and say, "I can eat that," without worrying too much about what its calorie content is. At the same time, you ought to be staying away from that fast food outlet, except for the occasional odd treat.

If weight loss is your goal, you should definitely focus on burning as many calories as you can to achieve your ideal weight. Take note that it is more important to eat calories from protein rather than from carbohydrates. Your body also converts protein into energy, and this allows you to burn fat while staying energetic. Reducing calorie intake is important, and for your reference, there are a number of calorie counters online that you can download or use to keep track of the amount of calories you eat in each meal or dish.

Also, remember to reduce the amount of calorie you consume from added sugars, as these typically cause weight gain. Added sugars are usually found in carbonated drinks, energy drinks, sports drinks, desserts, fruit drinks, and candy.

The best and most accurate way to burn calories is by working out. If you work out consistently, then you won't need to worry quite as much about how many calories you take in. This way, you can stick with just worrying about eating healthy rather than counting your calories. Of course, just because you are burning the calories you're eating doesn't mean that you can get away with eating anything that you want. In fact, it's the opposite. You'll need to make sure that you only eat healthier foods if you want a better chance of losing weight and being healthy.

On The Subject Of Sugar

Whilst we are here, it might be a good idea to take a look at some of the bad guys and how they got us into this mess in the first place. We will also look into how to avoid them. Over the next ten years, we will see the escalation of the war on added sugar, which is now recognized as a health threat on par with tobacco. The sugar industry is already starting to put up a fight to defend their business in much the same way that the tobacco industry did; only this time, they have been able to learn from the mistakes made by the big tobacco companies.

Experts now believe that sugar can easily become a complete addictive substance in much the same way as drugs are. In an experiment conducted by French scientists in Bordeaux, it was discovered that rats chose sugar rather than cocaine, even when they were addicted to cocaine.

Sugar was first cultivated by man on the island of New Guinea some 10 000 years ago. At that stage, it was simply picked and eaten raw. It gradually spread and is believed to have reached mainland Asia about 1000 B.C. It was carried by the conquering Arab caliphs, and as their power spread, sugar use spread, too. Once the British and French discovered it, demand soared, and the slave trade was born.

The reason I have touched briefly on the history of sugar is to show how recently it became a part of the human diet. In the 1700s, the average Englishman consumed four pounds per year. By 1800, that amount soared to eighteen pounds, but that was just the start. Come 1870, an English commoner would have been eating around forty-seven pounds per year, which then leapt to one hundred pounds per year in just thirty years. Today, the average American consumes seventy-seven pounds of added sugar.

What is the consequence of this colossal sugar addiction of ours? One-third of adults have high blood pressure, and three hundred and forty-seven million suffer from diabetes. Early nutrition experts who were first to start raising the alarm bell about the devastating effects of sugar on our health were simply drowned out by those blaming high cholesterol for the modern afflictions of obesity and heart disease. Over the last twenty years, fat consumption in the US has gone down, and yet, obesity levels are going up faster than ever.

American endocrinologist Robert Lustig says, "It has nothing to do with calories. Sugar is a poison by itself when consumed in high doses."

Here is the real catch: sugar is really difficult to avoid, especially if you eat fast food and ready meals, because it is an essential ingredient used by the food industry to add taste. Taste is even more necessary if the fat levels of meals have been lowered to persuade people that they are eating something healthy.

Lustig goes on to say, "An analysis of one hundred and seventy-five countries over the past decade showed that when you look for the cause of type 2 (non-insulin dependent) diabetes, the total number of calories you consume is irrelevant. It's the specific calories that count. When people ate one hundred and fifty calories every day, the rate of diabetes went up by 0.1 percent. However, if those calories came from a can of fizzy drink, the rate went up to 1.1 percent. Added sugar is eleven times more potent in causing diabetes than general calories." There are complicated scientific reasons for this, and the whole of science will be in dispute for years to come, but reducing sugar intake appears to be crucial not only for weight loss, but for overall health as well. The average 12-ounce can of soda contains ten teaspoons of sugar. If you consider that some people consume two or three such drinks during the course of a day, is it any wonder that obesity has reached the levels that it has?

When looking at foods to eat, it's pretty obvious that you should find the foods that have less sugar. Any foods that have no sugar added are even better. Anything that you might want to add sugar to should not have any sugar in the first place. This way, you won't be eating too much sugar.

The Role Of The Food Industries

As I have previously mentioned, the food industry plays a crucial role in what we eat. Between 1977 and 2000, sugar intake in the United States doubled, yet sales of granulated sugar remained the same or even dropped. In short, we have been getting our sugar somewhere else. Eighty percent of the food items for sale in the average supermarket contain added sugar. This may come in one or two different forms, but the most popular is high-fructose corn syrup.

It is the fructose in sugars that our bodies have a problem processing. When you eat an apple, it contains high quantities of fructose, but it is accompanied by fiber, such that it is processed via the stomach. Refined sugars are sent directly to the liver, which soon becomes overloaded and is forced to store those sugars as fat—most commonly, belly fat. With sugar estimated to be eight times more addictive than cocaine, we soon find ourselves in a position in which our craving for sugar skyrockets, and the vicious cycle begins. Our bodies store the sugar as fats. We become less energetic and move less, and as a result, we process the whole food we do eat less efficiently.

The US government has tried to reign in the food industry several times, but every time this happens, companies immediately cry "nanny state" or "government attack on our freedom to choose." These food giants have a huge amount of clout. They throw huge budgets at advertising campaigns promoting the health advantages of their products, yet they have firmly resisted giving clear labels as to how much sugar our supermarket products contain. In 1950, the first links to lung cancer were proven, but it took another fifty years of denial on the part of the tobacco industry before we began to see real change in the way cigarettes were marketed. This will be the first generation in the United States where children will have a shorter life expectancy than their parents did. Can we afford to wait another fifty years before we get a grip on the amount of additives in our food?

It All Starts With The Kids

A significant percentage of the food industry advertising budget is directed toward our children. After all, if you can hook them and cause them to become addicted while they are young, then chances are, companies will have a customer for life. The food that our children are served in school cafeterias is rarely of the quality that it should be, and the contracts to supply those cafeterias are normally held by big players in the industry. The ban on tobacco advertising resulted in a fifty percent reduction in high school smokers over twenty years. Is it not time that the advertising of high-sugar foods to our kids be banned as well? In fact, the legislation pertaining to advertising to children is not as strict as advertising to adults. It is in our children that we are seeing the fastest rise in obesity levels, particularly in poorer communities. Several attempts to ban or reduce advertising targeting young people have been overturned. The lobby groups in the food industry know where their long-term client base lies.

Type 2 diabetes used to be known as adult-onset diabetes, but that term became outdated when an increasing number of young children began to become obese. Doctors understand the methods used to treat diabetes in adults, but treating this new young and obese generation will take them into unchartered territory as they now begin treating people over nearly the entire course of their lives.

As parents, you should make sure to keep your kids as far from those unhealthy foods as possible. They can have candy every so often and have other things on occasion, but it should never be every day. Starting when they are very young, you should aim to have your kids eating healthy foods. It doesn't have to be the same five foods over and over again, but it does need to be foods that they will enjoy. Give them a huge variety of foods to try. Also, you should limit their exposure to ads on TV, especially when they are very young. This will keep their minds off of food that they might see on TV and only on the foods that you make them. They will be less tempted to try something unhealthy they saw if they never saw it in the first place.

So Where Do We Go From Here?

We may be marketed to very aggressively, but we can still choose to eat healthy foods if we want to. Most of the salt and sugar we eat come in the form of real food that is engineered. If we go back to real food, we suddenly find our sugar and salt levels dropping dramatically, and that is not to say anything about colorings and preservatives. The food industry would have us believe that buying real meat and vegetables is going to hurt our budgets, but considerable research is now proving that this is simply not true. Where food companies are at an advantage is that they sell convenience. Real food needs to be cooked or prepared in some way, whereas much of the prepared food we are sold simply needs to be popped into a microwave for a few minutes, and a lot of fast food does not even require that.

The single most powerful thing you can do to improve both your health and that of your family is to develop a passion for home cooking. Sure, you are busy, and you have had a hard day at work, but isn't the health of your family more important? During the course of this book, I will show you several ways to make home cooking easier and more fun. We will also give you some easy, quick-to-prepare recipes that are not only healthy, but can also be stored to warm up on those days when you simply don't want to spend a long time cooking. These are only examples, however, and this is not a cookbook. There are thousands of healthy eating cookbooks on the market, as well as dozens of programs on television. Why don't you try eliminating all processed food from your diet for just one week and see how much better you feel? Hopefully, after that, you will be on the road to continuing a healthy lifestyle.

Choose Macro-Nutrients

The literal definition of a macro-nutrient is any substance that a living organism needs in large quantities. Animals that are carnivores need more protein, since their diet is primarily meat. For omnivores, they have a plant based diet. Then, there are omnivores, like humans. They need a mix of both meat and plants to have a healthy diet. Therefore, the macro-nutrients that an omnivore needs will be much more than the others, since they need a mix of plants and meat. Dogs are another example of an omnivore, as their diet is a mix of plants and meat. However, they can't be deprived of meat, even if they are an omnivore. This can cause many issues in their body, as the food they should be eating needs to have a balance. Cats, however, are much more carnivores. They can't go without eating meat, as they need more meat to survive than any other food.

Simply put, macro-nutrients are a combination of fat, protein, and carbohydrates. If you are trying to lose weight, it is important that you eat 1 to 1.5 grams of protein, less than a gram of carbohydrates, and around 0.5 to 2.5 grams of fat per pound of your bodyweight per day. As an example, someone weighing 150 lbs would need to eat 150 to 225 grams of protein, less than 150 grams of carbohydrates, and between 75 and 375 grams of fat each day.

Go Easy On Sodium

Salt is another of those additives that are eating way too much of for our own good, but most of what we do eat does not come from that small quantity we choose to sprinkle over our meals. It is recommended that we consume no more than 2.3

milligrams of salt per day. In the US, the average daily intake is 3.4 milligrams. This excessive intake can lead to high blood pressure, stroke, osteoporosis, and even asthma.

Sodium, as you might guess, holds more liquid in your body. This, in turn, causes a lot of strain on your heart, making it possible for you to suffer from a heart attack. Along with the heart, it can also damage the aorta, which is the major artery into your heart, the kidneys, and also the bones. An increase in your sodium intake might not make your blood pressure go up, but that doesn't mean you're in the clear. There are many other issues that can arise from a huge amount of salt intake.

In the United Kingdom alone, it is estimated that eighty-five percent of our daily salt intake comes from that added by the food industry. In the United States, similar figures are showing up. The food industry knows that we like the taste of salt, and they are out to make sure we don't lose the taste for it either.

Here are a few common food items that add to the excess salt we are consuming:

Bread: ½ gram per slice

Biscuits: ½ gram per two biscuits

Canned: soup 3 grams

Pizza: 2.5 grams

Many processed meats are high in sodium, and those same products have now been found to have strong links to cancer. It is important to read labels to see how much sodium you are about to buy, but the best choice are those labels that say sodium-free. You can then add your own salt according to your own taste and in quantities that you know are healthy. Our taste buds are conditioned to high quantities of salt, which is why we like fast food so much. It is possible to wean yourself off of salt, just do it gradually. To give food a little bit of extra taste, try adding dried herbs, curry, or ginger.

Some great specific spices or dried herbs to add to your dishes includes basil, thyme, cumin, chili powder, rosemary, red pepper flakes, cinnamon, and oregano. Basil is more frequently put in pasta sauces. It has a great flavor that will definitely bring out the Italian flavor you might want in your pasta. Thyme is often seen as a flavoring on fish fillets, but it also is frequently smothered on chicken. It has a bit of an earthy taste to it and can really make your dish stand out. Cumin is used in a lot of different foods, including chicken, ground meat, and vegetables. If you're a big chili lover, then you've found the perfect thing to add to your chili dish to make it the best it can be.

Chili powder is frequently paired with cumin in a dish. Of course, you'll be putting chili powder in chili. It wouldn't really be chili without it. It gives any dish a nice little kick, so if you ever have a dish that you want to have some heat, sprinkle some chili powder in. Rosemary is a great dried herb to use just before grilling or roasting some meat and potatoes. It is frequently seen in potatoes, especially roasted potatoes. Red pepper flakes are in the same vein as chili powder. If you want a little kick in your dish, you might decide that red pepper flakes are the way to go. If you get a bite with a red pepper flake in it, you'll know. This is also a great spice to add to any spice rub, as long as you want a little heat. Plus, you don't need to go overboard to get that kick you're looking for.

Cinnamon might seem like a strange choice for some people, but it can be that little sweetener you've been looking for. It doesn't even need to be something super exciting. You can use it in some yogurt to give it some flavor, especially if you have some plain vanilla Greek yogurt. Add some fruit chunks and you've got a great snack food. Adding cinnamon to a savory dish is also possible. Maybe you want to make some spaghetti that has a little bit of a sweet side. Sprinkle a little cinnamon in and notice the change. Finally, there is oregano, which is another great Italian dish herb. Adding some oregano to any pasta dish will work out and make it taste even better. Garlic bread can always use some oregano and the same goes with some vegetables, especially if you're having an Italian styled dinner.

It's Okay To Eat Fat

If there is one food source that has been given a bad rap over the last thirty or forty years, it has to be fat. Sure, too much of the wrong fats—too much of any fat for that matter—can be bad for you, but fat is not the big bad guy it has been made out to be. We have been fed decades of anti-fat, low-fat, and fat-free propaganda over the years. Much of that propaganda comes via the food industry that discovered a neat little trick. Knock out the fat, add sugar to give the food some taste, and sell it back to consumers at a higher price as a healthy alternative. The fact of the matter is that we need fat in our diet. Fat provides us with essential fatty acids, helps keep our skin soft, and provides fat-soluble vitamins. More importantly, fat provides us with energy. Somehow, we have bought into the notion that eating fat and being fat amount to the same thing. We cannot function for more than a few days without eating fat. Humans have been eating fats for a lot longer than they have been eating carbohydrates, for example, and they have always been lean. It is only the last few decades that there has been a sudden growth in our waistlines. Until recently, the argument has been that the massive global weight gains we have seen came about because of the failure to control our willpower, and the assumption is that if we simply retake control of that willpower, we will become thin again. Anyone who has ever tried to diet and then maintain the weight loss will soon tell you that it is not quite that easy. Something has gone wrong somewhere with the way we eat, and simple self-control is not the answer.

Let's take a look at the appestat. The appestat is a part of the human brain believed to control body weight. In short, this small part of our anatomy controls appetite, and it does so by regulating food intake. That appestat is sated by clean healthy fats, but it becomes confused when exposed to fats and sugars in processed food that provide calories but no nutrients. In short, it is looking for nutrients, and when it does not find any or does not find enough, you remain hungry. That is why it is so difficult to eat just one chocolate cookie or one potato chip.

As long as you're eating the right kinds of fat, then there's nothing wrong with it. Mono-saturated and poly-saturated fats are both good fats, and you should eat foods that are rich in them. Fat is actually an energy source that is good for your body, especially in the absence or reduction of carbohydrates. Fats also make up cell membranes and are important in the regeneration or reproduction of cells, as well as in muscle and joint recovery. The best kinds of fat include those that are full of Omega-3 and Omega-6 acids, such as tuna and salmon, because they activate your body's fat-burning genes and give your body better fat storage.

You should take note that around 10% of your daily calorie intake must come from fats. This will be easy because full-fat dairy products, peanut butter, and most animal products all have good fats in them. More examples of foods rich in good fats can be found on the chart below:

Mono-Saturated Fats	Canola Oil, Olive Oil, Peanut Oil, Sunflower Oil, Olives, Avocados, Peanut Butter, Hazelnut, Cashews, Pecans, Macadamia Nuts, Almonds
Poly-Saturated Fats	Corn Oil, Soybean Oil, Walnuts, Safflower Oil, Flax seed, Tuna, Salmon, Mackerel, Sardines, Trout, Herring

Meanwhile, some examples of bad fats include:

Saturated Fats	Chicken with skin, High-fat portions of beef chicken, or pork, Cheese, Butter, Ice cream, Lard, Palm oil, Coconut oil
Trans Fats	Chips, Packaged popcorn, Crackers, Commercially baked doughnuts, Pastries, Cakes, Muffins, Pizza dough, Vegetable shortening, Stick margarine, Candy bars, French fries, Chicken nuggets, Fried chicken, Breaded fish

It's Okay To Have A Cheat Day

Leptin is something that is produced by your fat cells. When your leptin levels are sufficient for the amount of energy you need, then your brain will be signaled, telling you that you don't need to eat anymore. It's a little different when you are dieting. Many diets restrict calories. This means that every day, you are restricting your body from the leptin that it needs. Your body won't think you are getting the energy that you need for proper survival, so it can cause you to have a day where you eat a lot more than you should, also known as binging. Even if you've been eating a good amount of food and getting the nutrients you need, your leptin levels might not be where they should be. However, if you have a cheat day once a week, then you won't have to worry about a time in the future where you will be uncontrollably binging.

If you allow yourself a day of eating burgers, fries, pizza, and chocolate, you'll be keener on making sure that you eat clean again the following days. Just be sure you don't go overboard with the amount of calories you consume. Having a cheat day will also burn more calories by boosting your metabolism. This is due to your thyroid hormones. The more that you restrict calories, the slower your metabolism will go. With a slower metabolism, the chances of losing weight start to go way down. This cheat day might be exactly what your body needs to keep going and losing weight. As long as you are eating clean throughout the week, this increase in calories will actually burn fat and have you looking forward to the next cheat day again. Remember to do this only once each week!

Don't Starve Yourself

Skipping meals to lose weight does not work! Some people think that if they skip meals, then they are helping themselves lose weight faster. The thing is, if you skip meals or starve yourself, you're actually slowing down your metabolism, which means that your body stores fat rather than burning it. If your body doesn't know when its next meal is coming, it will hold on to the fat it has in case energy is needed. Starving yourself has no fat loss benefits and is not healthy in any way, so just don't do it.

Doing this a few times might make you think that you're losing weight, but you really aren't. It can lead to anorexia or any other combination of these types of eating disorders. Also, the more that your body doesn't get the nutrients it needs, the more likely it might start breaking down the muscle in your body to give it some energy. Not eating only leads to issues with your body, it doesn't help you lose weight in a healthy way.

Know More About The Glycemic Index

The glycemic index is a means of measuring the effect of carbohydrates on blood sugar levels. It's important to eat foods with low glycemic index because these foods keep your blood sugar levels balanced. Moreover, the body is able to burn these foods efficiently to give you the right amount of energy. Meanwhile, foods with high glycemic index spike your blood sugar levels, thus causing your body to go into a fat storing phase. These are the foods you want to avoid. Take a look at the chart below, which provides a sample of commonly eaten foods:

Low GI (less than 55)	Apple, Broccoli, Cherries, Grapefruit, Orange, Pear, Tomatoes
Medium GI (56 to 69)	Banana, Brown Rice, Oatmeal, Popcorn, Sweet Potato, White Rice, Whole Wheat Bread
High GI (70 and up)	Bagel, Doughnuts, Rice Cakes, Pretzels, Watermelon, White Bread, White Potatoes

Read Nutrition Labels

It's extremely important to read nutrition labels or "nutrition facts" on food packages. Understanding what makes up the food that you eat is important. Knowing if you are eating the right amount of nutrients or if what you've bought is high in calories or high in sodium is extremely helpful. Knowing how to read nutrition labels will go a long way in helping you reach your weight loss goals. In the next chapter, you will learn more about reading nutrition labels.

Nicholas Bjorn

Chapter 3: Reading Nutrition Labels

Reading nutrition labels is not only good for yourself and your own needs, but also good when you are cooking for other people. If you know someone is gluten free, you'll need to make sure you get something without any gluten. The same goes for anyone who might have a food allergy, as those are stated around the ingredients list just below the nutrition label on most food packages. This is also helpful when you are looking at food for your pets. The labels aren't exactly the same, but knowing how to read a regular nutrition label can still help.

Here's what you need to know about reading Nutrition Labels:

Number Of Servings And Serving Sizes

Take note that nutritional facts are mostly based on one serving only. Always check the serving size to know how many servings you are going to consume. This means that the bigger the serving, the higher the calories.

Along with that, you need to know how many servings would be approximately how much you would be consuming. Take a bag of chips, for example. Usually at the top of the label, it will tell you how many chips make up a single serving. From there, you'll know just how much sodium you'll be eating from a serving size of eleven chips, for example. Most people eat more than eleven chips, of course, but you can still get a general idea of how much sodium you'll be consuming with how many chips you are eating.

When you are comparing nutrients and calories between two different food brands, always review the serving sizes to ensure that they are based on the same measurement. Many brands will have slightly different serving sizes, but as long as you are comparing two things that are the same, you should get a good idea of the differences in nutrition.

Pay Attention To The Amount Of Calories

The "Calories" label under "Amount per Serving" is where you will see the number of calories the product has per serving. You'll also see the amount of calories from fat here.

Take note that even if something is fat-free, it doesn't mean that it's also free from calories. Even if a product is low-fat, it may have the same amount of calories as other products have, so always check the number of calories in the label.

One thing to keep in mind is that just because something has a lot of calories, it doesn't mean that you are eating badly. You should be more concerned with how many of those calories come from fat. If a lot of the calories are from fat, then you might want to steer clear of that product. Or, you could see if another brand has that product with less calories from fat. Then, you'll still be able to get the food you want, but it will be a lot better for you.

Calories are not inherently bad. What is bad is consuming too many calories every day and not burning enough of them off. If you mix that with a lot of calories from fat, you might notice some weight staying on your body. If, however, you work out regularly, you can get away with eating things that have a lot of calories. Of course, you also need to balance that out with eating healthy things as well, since you can't quickly and easily lose weight by eating junk all the time, no matter how much you work out.

As an example, a product lists that there are 100 calories per 3 candy bars. This means that when you eat 6 candy bars, you consumed 2 servings, and thus, you have consumed twice the amount of calories.

The %Dv Is Your Friend

%DV or the percentage of Dietary Value that each nutrient gives is essential for you to know how much of each nutrient you should consume daily to live a healthy life. If you want to you this most effectively, you'll need to make sure that you record all the %DV that you consume of each a day. If any nutrients go over 100, then you'll know you're consuming more than you need to. You should try to keep it as close to one hundred as possible.

This is also a great way to find out if you're not consuming enough of any particular nutrient. Anemia is very common and can be prevented by making sure you're taking in enough iron. If you are consistently not consuming very much every day, you should find ways to add to it. There are plenty of foods that can help you take in more iron every day. Just to make sure that you are, be sure to look at the nutrition label!

Look For Products That Are Rich In Calcium, Iron, And Vitamins A And C

Most adults do not get enough of these vitamins and minerals through their daily food consumption. It would be extremely beneficial if you choose products that are rich in these vitamins and minerals. The best way to make sure you are getting enough is by simply finding foods that have a good mix of these. There are tons of foods out there you can find that can give you everything you need, so make sure to look at the nutrition labels.

Choose Good Fats

Again, it's alright to consume fats just as long as they are the right kinds of fats. Choose foods that are low in cholesterol, saturated fat, and trans fat. As often as possible, replace saturated fat with mono or poly-saturated fats to lower your blood cholesterol levels.

Some products list trans-fat as having 0% Dietary Value, but it would be best to consume only a little or truly eliminate it from your diet because trans-fat lowers the amount of good cholesterol, which makes you susceptible to heart diseases.

Take note that the Dietary Value Percentage (%DV) for total fat is the computation of all the kinds of fat in one product.

Check The Sodium Count

This is definitely an important thing to check. A lot of foods have salt that's been already added in and some foods can have a ton of salt. For the average adult, they should be consuming no more than 2,300 milligrams a day. Some packaged foods can have over 1,000 milligrams in them already, especially if it's a frozen dinner type food. Therefore, you should find lower sodium foods by not only making your own dinners from scratch, but also cutting out the canned and processed foods as much as possible.

Some foods like that have the sodium count on the front of the package, so you might not even have to look specifically at the nutrition label to find what you need. At the same time, it's always helpful to look at that label anyway. You might find that it's not as bad as you originally thought.

Weight Management

It might not come as much of a shock, but knowing how to read nutrition labels can help you maintain your weight. If you keep track of how much saturated and trans fat you are eating every day, this can help you lessen your fat intake. Also, you can also find exactly what foods you need to eat in order to lose weight in the most effective way. Foods high in nutrients and low in fat and calories are great foods to eat.

Even though calorie counting is the way most people know how to go on a diet, it really is not very effective. Eating something low in calories doesn't mean you are eating healthy. When you think about it, something could have very little calories, but a lot of those calories are from fat. However, eating a proper diet that is a mixture of all the good things you need will ensure better results.

Go For Healthy Carbohydrates

Remember that fiber and sugar are also carbohydrate sources. Fruits, vegetables, whole grains, and beans are carbohydrates, but they are good in reducing the risk of heart disease. Plus, they improve the way your digestive system works.

You'll know that something is considered "whole" or is part of the "whole foods" group if it says so in the ingredient list. Examples include whole oats, whole wheat rice, and whole wheat bread.

While there is no %DV for sugar, you can check how much sugar there is in one product by comparing it with other brands and looking for "sugar content."

Try to limit your intake of foods that include added sugars. Examples of added sugars include corn syrup, fructose, glucose, maple syrup, and sucrose. All these sugars do is add calories to your diet without adding any nutritional benefits.

You might notice that there are very few foods now that don't have corn syrup in some capacity. High fructose corn syrup is in many different foods because it's cheap to make and an easy additive in a food. However, that doesn't mean it's healthy.

High fructose corn syrup is a variation of sugar, but it is much sweeter. It is also in a lot of foods at a higher amount than regular sugar usually is. Look at any label of a food that has this additive and you'll notice that many times, it is the very first ingredient. Sugar in large amounts is already very unhealthy, so having something like this is almost worse. Since it is in so many different foods, trying to find foods without it is hard. Though it would be better to go without, a good first step is finding the foods where it is not the first ingredient, but lower down on the ingredient list.

Protein May Be Essential, But You Should Still Go For Low-Fat

Always choose products that are lean, fat-free, or low-fat to be able to maximize protein intake and to ensure that fats are burned or converted into energy. When you take a piece of chicken, there shouldn't be very much fat on the chicken itself if it is low fat or lean. It's very easy to tell on chicken, since the fat is white. If it is a meat where you can easily see the fat, then you should make sure to look at it before you purchase it.

Steak is a wonderful source of protein, but not all steak cuts are the same. Some of them will have a lot more fat than others. The leanest cuts include various round cuts and top sirloin. You can always double check on any cut of steak by seeing if there is a lot of white fat on it. The less, the better.

For something like chicken, it's best to go without the skin. The skin holds a lot of fat, so it isn't the best idea to eat when you are trying to lose weight. Even if you can't buy the skinless chicken, you can always take the skins off before you cook it. Also, the healthiest part of the chicken is the breast, so try to get skinless chicken breasts if you can.

Keep these things in mind to make better, healthier choices the next time you visit your grocery store.

Nicholas Bjorn

Chapter 4: The Right Vitamins And Minerals

Aside from keeping the foods mentioned earlier in mind, take note that in order to lose weight while still feeling energetic, you need to consume foods that are rich in the right kinds of vitamins and minerals. In this chapter, you will learn more about these substances.

Vitamin A

Vitamin A is important in helping you maintain normal vision and in keeping the eyes, teeth, skin, and skeletal system healthy. It also helps regenerate cells and tissues that will enable you to live a better and healthier life.

Vitamin A is also crucial in keeping your immune system strong and healthy. It is a regulator for many of the genes that work to fight of things as simple as colds, but also things like cancer. If you are deficient in vitamin A, you'll likely notice that you are sick a lot more often than other people who are consuming enough of this vitamin.

This can also help reduce the chances of some food allergies. It is a natural anti-inflammatory, one that specifically effects the inflammation that occurs during a food allergy. While this can't reverse the effects of a food allergy, it might prevent some allergies from occurring. It has also been seen to reduce the chances of a degenerative disease like Alzheimer's or Parkinson's.

Examples of foods rich in Vitamin A include:

- Baked Eel
- Beef Liver
- Skimmed Milk
- Pickled Herring
- Goat Cheese
- 1 Large Egg
- Salmon
- Canned Pumpkin
- Sweet Potato
- Chopped Raw Kale
- Raw Carrots
- Spinach
- Butternut Squash
- Raw Cantaloupe
- Dried Apricots
- Cooked Spinach

Vitamin B6

Vitamin B6 is essential in producing enzymes that convert protein into energy to help you lose weight quickly. It also helps you maintain normal red and white blood cell levels, as well as reduces the risk of heart disease and anemia. Vitamin B6 likewise synthesizes neurotransmitters that are responsible for carrying brain signals from one nerve to the other.

This also acts as a natural pain treatment, specifically for fibroids in the uterus, which can be incredibly painful. Many B vitamins are useful in making this pain much more manageable. It can also be used to help boost your mood. It helps stimulate the growth of serotonin and norepinephrine, which are two hormones that help boost your mood. Finally, Vitamin B6 can also create antibodies, which help fight off many different illnesses that you might experience.

You might notice a deficiency if you've noticed a change in your mood towards irritability, anxiety, or depression, had a lack of energy, confusion, worsening PMS symptoms, muscle pains, or confusion. These things won't happen instantly, but if you notice many of these things happening, then you should definitely see if you are deficient in Vitamin B6.

Foods rich in Vitamin B6 include:

- All Bran Cereal

- Yellow Fin Tuna

- Soy-Based Vegetarian Meat

- Canned Tuna

- Sunflower Seeds

- Chicken Or Turkey Liver

- Boneless And Skinless Chicken Breast

- 1 Medium Banana

- Cooked Venison

- Cooked Salmon

- Cooked Trout

- Cooked Lentils

- Baked Potato (Skin Intact)

- Chopped Red Bell Pepper

- Cooked Chickpeas

- Instant Cooked Oatmeal

Vitamin B12

Vitamin B12 is also responsible for converting protein and fats into energy, which can be used in ensuring that the skin, eyes, and teeth are healthy. It is also essential in ensuring the health of nerve cells and in producing genetic material, such as DNA. It is used as a protective cover on the nerves, keeping them from harm as much as possible.

Vitamin B12 is also important in digestion and heart health. The amino acid homocysteine is regulated by how much Vitamin B12 is in your system. This amino acid, when the levels are elevated, can be dangerous, so keeping them in check with Vitamin B12 is important.

Vitamin B12 is also important in making sure a pregnancy is healthy and goes without any issues. Since it is a building block for DNA, it makes sense that a deficiency in Vitamin B12 can cause a pregnancy to not work properly.

Foods rich in Vitamin B12 include:

- Cooked Beef Liver

- Canned Sardines

- Cooked Mackerel

- Black Or Red Caviar

- Cooked Pork Kidney

- 1 Cup Soy Beverage

- 1 Bran Raisin Cereal

- 1 Cup Cottage Cheese

- 3 Oz Ground Beef

- 1 Cup Skimmed Milk

- 3 Oz Cooked Ham

- 1 Cup Homo Milk

- 1 Cup Plain Yogurt

- Soy-Based Vegetarian Meat

Vitamin C

Vitamin C is often regarded as one of the most important nutrients for the human body. It is used in so many different aspects of your body and is crucial in your overall health. There have actually been studies done to suggest that the amount you should be getting daily is higher than what you might physically be able to get. You can't eat the amount of fruits and vegetables that you would need every day that would bring your vitamin C levels up to where they should be. Therefore, if you want to get the full benefits of Vitamin C, it would be best to take a daily supplement that would bring you up to 500 milligrams a day.

This is a great anti-oxidant, which means that it helps in the production and regeneration of cells. It also helps in making your skin look beautiful and gives you that radiant glow. It is essential in the anti-aging process, and it has great anti-inflammatory benefits that help protect you against cold, cough, and flu. You definitely want to make sure you're getting enough Vitamin C if you want to fight off any illnesses you might have. It is important in the proper development of your bones, gums, and blood vessels. It is also a crucial vitamin for prenatal development, so any expecting mothers should make sure they have plenty of vitamin C in their bodies.

Examples of foods rich in Vitamin C include:

- Broccoli

- ½ Cup Guava

- ½ Cup Sliced Kiwi

- Red Raw Bell Peppers, Chopped

- Green Raw Bell Peppers, Chopped

- ½ Cup Mashed Papaya

- ½ Cup Lychee

- 4 Sprouts Brussels Sprouts Cooked

- ½ Grapefruit

- ½ Cup Navel Orange

- ½ Cup Sliced Strawberries

- ½ Cup Red

- Raw Cabbage

- ½ Cup Pineapple Chunks

Vitamin D

Vitamin D works mainly for the proper growth of bones and teeth. It also regulates calcium and phosphate levels in the blood and helps maintain proper cell growth and neuro-muscular function. With the calcium and phosphate levels, this helps maintain proper immune system functions. With the proper amount of Vitamin D, you can have more protection against certain diseases.

If you don't get the proper amount of Vitamin D and are deficient, it can lead to issues like soft or fragile bones (osteomalacia or osteoporosis). However, it can also protect you from diseases like multiple sclerosis and heart disease. If you have depression, Vitamin D might alleviate some of your symptoms. It has been shown to help regulate your mood, which helps with depression and anxiety.

As for weight loss, there have been a few studies done to see if Vitamin D can help in any way. In one study, those taking the Vitamin D saw a small amount of weight loss, but it wasn't anything significant. Another study gave a group both Vitamin D and calcium. This group had more significant results, as the mix of Vitamin D and calcium seemed to have an appetite repressing effect. Overall, Vitamin D is an important vitamin that you need plenty of.

Foods rich in Vitamin D include:

- 1 Can Tuna, Drained

- Baked Salmon

- 1 Cup Cow's Milk

- 2 Pieces Pacific Sardines, In Tomato Sauce

- Soy or Almond Milk

- Low-Fat Yogurt

- 1 Cup Orange Juice

- 1 Tbsp. Margarine

- 1 Large Egg

- 1 Cup Breakfast Cereal

- 1 Cup Raw Mushroom Slices

Vitamin E

Vitamin E is a great anti-oxidant that protects the body from being damaged by free radicals to prevent disease and cancer. It also protects the skin from ultraviolet rays that cause skin damage and skin cancer.

If you have had high cholesterol or come from a family that generally has high cholesterol, you might consider upping your intake of Vitamin E. It has a balancing effect and stops the cholesterol from oxidizing, which is what makes it go higher.

Since it fights inflammation, it is a great natural way to boost your immune system. Also, it is a natural anti-aging nutrient. It can protect your skin from premature wrinkles and any damage that you might get throughout the years. Along with that, it can help heal your skin from sunburns, scars, and acne. If you've always had naturally thin hair, consuming more Vitamin E might help thicken it, giving you the thick hair you've always wanted. It can also help keep your scalp from getting dry and flakey, something many people have to deal with, especially in the winter.

Vitamin E is a natural hormone balancer. It can help regulate your menstrual period, especially if it is being addled by your hormones. Another hormonal imbalance might cause you to have unnecessary weight gain. This can be especially stressful, but having a good amount of Vitamin E might change that, making it possible to regulate your weight instead of it regulating you.

Examples of foods rich in Vitamin E are as follows:

- ¼ Cup Peanuts

- ¼ Cup Almonds

- ¼ Cup Sunflower Seeds

- 1 Tsp Wheat Germ Oil

- 2 Tbsp Almond Butter

- ½ Cup Canned Tomato Sauce

- ½ Cup Cooked Spinach

- ¼ Cup Pine Nuts

- ¼ Cup Toasted Wheat Germ Cereal

- ½ Cup Cooked Turnip Greens

- ½ Cup Cooked Swiss Chard

- 1 Tsp Sunflower Oil

Vitamin K

Vitamin K helps in synthesizing proteins so they can be used as energy. This also helps burn fat. Vitamin K prevents blood clots. Of course, this doesn't mean that it never allows your blood to clot. It regulates it to clot when it needs to and make sure that you don't have any sort of bad blood clot, like a stroke. Along with this, Vitamin K is essential in building strong bones.

It is crucial in preventing the calcification of arteries and other soft tissues. This is when calcium builds up in places where it isn't supposed to be. While some of this calcification is normal, not all of it is. It can cause major issues in some cases, disrupting normal organ functions and getting in the way of blood vessels. Vitamin K can help regulate this and stop this from happening in places that it shouldn't.

A Vitamin K deficiency can lead to defective blood clotting, increased bleeding, and osteoporosis. This blood clotting might be more severe or might not happen at all. If it doesn't happen, you might bleed too much. The opposite can also occur, which can cause a number of different issues.

There are three different types of Vitamin K. K1 and K2 have been shown to be the most effective at preventing certain cancers. K2 seems to be the most effective with most of the issues Vitamin K takes care of, including protection against heart disease and osteoporosis. K3 is not a recommended vitamin. It has shown to have some levels of toxicity and should be avoided.

Foods rich in Vitamin K include:

- 1 Cup Raw Turnip Greens

- ½ Cup Cooked Brussels Sprouts

- 1 Cup Raw Swiss Chard

- ½ Cup Raw Parsley

- 1 Cup Raw Kale

- 1 Tbsp. Canola Oil

- ½ Cup Raw Scallions

- 1 Tbsp. Soybean Oil

- 1 Cup Raw Romaine Lettuce

- ½ Cup Raw Broccoli

- ½ Cup Raw Scallions

- 1 Cup Raw Collard Greens

Calcium

While it may be fully regulated in the body, it is still important that you make calcium a part of your diet to ensure the proper health of bones and teeth. It is especially important for strengthening your spine, as your spine is crucial for having a proper and proportionate body shape. It can keep your back from having pain as well, since it will be nice and strengthened. Calcium promotes proper muscle function and hormone secretion, which is why it's so important. This is especially true when it comes to the heart. Making sure your heart is strong and functioning well means that you won't have any issues with your heart. Having weak heart muscles is the last thing you want.

When paired with Vitamin D, calcium can have an effect on your weight. Having the proper amount of both in your body can help regulate your weight gain and help you lose weight easier. Calcium alone can do some of the work, but it's better when both are working at it. One big thing calcium does is prevent colon cancer. It suppresses the growth of polyps, which lead to the cancer. It has been shown to bind to the cancer promoters when going through your bowels and secreting them with it.

While kidney stones are calcium based, consuming calcium doesn't necessarily lead to kidney stones. In fact, having a good amount of calcium in your body might help prevent these kidney stones from forming. That, along with adequate water intake might stop any kidney stones from ever appearing.

Foods rich in calcium include:

- 6 Oz Plain Yogurt

- 6 Oz Fruit-Flavored Yogurt

- ½ Cup Cream Cheese

- ½ Cup Mozzarella Cheese

- 3 Oz Atlantic Sardines

- 3 Oz Pacific Sardines

- 1 Cup Nonfat Milk

- 1 Cup Reduced Fat Milk

- 1 Cup Skimmed Milk

- Soy or Nut Milk

- 3 Tbsp. Sesame Seeds

- 1 Cup Cooked Collard Greens

- ½ Cup Firm Tofu

- 1 Cup Frozen Spinach

- 1 Cup Boiled Mustard Greens

Iron

Iron helps muscles transport oxygen so that it can be used by the body. 70% of the iron in your body is found in hemoglobin, which is what transfers oxygen throughout your body. Not having enough iron is definitely not something you want to have, especially when it is used for something so important. It is also essential in helping increase your metabolism. The lack of iron may cause anemia, some symptoms of which are fatigue, energy loss, and shortness of breath. If you often have these symptoms, you may need to increase iron in your diet.

Without iron, we wouldn't have hemoglobin. This, of course, would mean that our entire bodies wouldn't be getting any oxygen, which is the last thing you would want. Along with that, we wouldn't have any muscles. Iron is crucial in muscle formation and is found in myoglobin, which is a muscle protein. It would be a very strange thing if we didn't have any muscles in our body, that's for sure.

Foods rich in iron are as follows:

- 1 Cup Whole Grain Breakfast Cereal

- 3 Oz Clams

- ¾ Cup Firm Tofu

- ¼ Cup Pumpkin Seeds

- 3 Oz Oysters

- 1 Tbsp. Molasses

- 1 Cup Prune Juice

- 3 Oz Beef

- 3 Oz Lamb Chops

- ¾ Cups Red Kidney Beans

- ¾ Cups Cooked Lentils

Potassium

Potassium is crucial in helping maintain electrolyte and water levels in the body and in ensuring that the heart, nervous system, and muscles all work well. The good news is that potassium is present in almost all plant and animal foods, as well as in unprocessed grains, milk, and legumes.

Having a high potassium intake is actually linked to a 20% reduced risk of dying from any number of deaths. It lowers the risk of things like a stroke. It is most primarily linked to blood pressure, since it lowers high blood pressure. It counteracts the effects of sodium, so you won't have to worry as much about having high blood pressure. Every organ in your body is kept in good condition thanks to potassium.

Here are some natural food sources of potassium:

- Bananas

- Avocados

- Almonds

- Peanuts

- Citrus Fruits

- Leafy Green Vegetables

- Milk

- Potatoes

Fiber

Fiber is incredibly important for your body. It helps with digestion, since fiber is actually something the body can't naturally digest. This helps make you feel full for longer and stops you from eating as much. Other benefits of fiber include blood sugar control and heart health. For anyone who has diabetes, you'll understand how important it is to regulate your blood sugar. Having a good amount of fiber can help your body do just that. Of course, even if you don't have diabetes, you should still be aware of this and actively try to keep your blood sugar levels at normal. Fiber also plays a significant role in your heart health. If you want to avoid having a heart attack or heart disease, then make sure you have the recommended amount of fiber in your body at all times.

Anyone who suffers from IBS will be glad to know that fiber also helps alleviate some of those symptoms. This has to do with the digestion aspects of fiber, namely that it is hard to digest. Having a good amount of fiber is also helpful for skin health. It has been linked to stopping certain skin ailments, such as acne, and making them much less severe. It works by moving yeast and fungus out of your body instead of it going through your pores. Your pores can't get clogged up, so you can't have acne. The risk of stroke is also decreased with the more fiber you eat. If your family has a history of strokes, you can help decrease that possibility by making sure to eat enough fiber.

For weight loss, fiber has been proven to be a great help. Also because of the digestion aspect of fiber, since it helps keep you feeling full for longer, you won't feel the need to go and grab an unhealthy snack. Instead, you can get through the day without worrying about snacking. If you do feel a little bit hungry, you can opt to grab something like nuts instead, which also add to the staving off of hunger. Things like hemorrhoids and kidney/gall stones are also going to be less common if you eat plenty of fiber. There are tons of great things that fiber can do, so you should always aim to get the recommended intake of fiber.

Here are a few foods with plenty of fiber:

- Carrots

- Avocados

- Berries

- Peas

- Almonds

- Oats

- Apples

- Bran Flakes

All of these vitamins and minerals are incredibly important for your body. Each one of them works in a different way, but they all work together to keep your body working properly. Without every single one of these vitamins and minerals, you would not be able to properly function. Your heart wouldn't have the things it needs to properly function and could even give out due to lack of muscle strength. You would be at a higher risk for numerous diseases, some of which have a high mortality rate.

There are even more vitamins and minerals that your body needs, but these ones are the most crucial ones. Be sure to look up the daily recommended consumption of all the nutrients not only on this list, but also the ones that aren't listed. All of these will help you get you the body you deserve to have, one that's healthy and strong.

Chapter 5: The Best Fat-Burning Foods

The road to weight loss can be incredibly frustrating. There will be foods you eat that might claim to help people lose weight, but just don't work for you at all. There are some foods out there that have been linked to helping people lose weight naturally, without taking any supplements. Of course, even if you do eat all of these foods, you'll still need to work out on top of this. As long as you have a set workout schedule and stick to it, you shouldn't have any problems with losing weight. If you want to you lose weight naturally as fast as possible, then you need to get to know the foods that burn fat faster than anything else. These foods are:

Walnuts

Walnuts contain Omega-3 Fatty Acids, one of the best kinds of fat out there. This provides the body with Alpha-Linolenic acid, which makes use of fats as energy and ensures that you are able to lose unnecessary fat. Eating a handful of every day will help you lose the weight you've been trying to lose. Even though walnuts are higher in fat and calories, that doesn't mean that it isn't incredibly healthy and can't help you lose weight. In some cases, it's proven to be more effective than a low fat diet, which is completely astonishing. What's even better about this is that you also can lower your cholesterol by eating walnuts every day. This is incredibly beneficial, especially when you are on your weight loss journey.

Water

A lot of people shrug off water and don't drink the amount they should. Some people just don't like the lack of taste while others just don't see the point. Water, however, is probably one of the most beneficial things you can do for your body. After all, the human body is made up of around 60% water, so it makes sense that drinking plenty of water will only help you. Water is necessary for your blood to keep flowing. Not having enough water can lead to dehydration, which is very bad for you. You will become fatigued, dizzy, confused, weak, and might even faint. However, if you drink the recommended amount of water daily, you'll be more than okay.

Drinking at least 2 cups of cold water increases your metabolic levels by around 30%, which means that it's one of the best things you can do to help reduce body fat. Water also keeps you hydrated and full of energy, which is important for you to get through each day. Drinking cold water is the best because your body will have to warm it up, which might burn some calories. Every extra calorie you can burn when trying to lose weight is helpful. Also, drinking while working out not only keeps you hydrated, but also can give your body that extra thing to do in order to lose weight.

Oatmeal

Aside from keeping blood sugar levels low, eating oatmeal boosts your metabolism. This makes sure that the body easily absorbs nutrients and that fat gets burned. Research shows that athletes who consume oatmeal in the mornings are able to burn more fat throughout the day than those who don't. What's even better about oatmeal is that you can use it for a variety of things you might cook. For example, you can use it to make something like banana bread. It will still have the great taste of banana bread, but will be much healthier. You could even use it as a substitute for breading on chicken, if you wanted to.

Oatmeal is also very low in fat. This makes it perfect for cutting down on the calories you're taking in every day. The fat that is in it is heart-healthy, mono and polyunsaturated fats. Another great thing about this is that it is a very filling food, making it a great breakfast item. You won't get as hungry throughout the day, so you won't overeat during lunch, which is likely your next meal.

Ginger

Ginger is great in making sure that the digestive system works well and that the digestive tract is clean. Ginger also reduces inflammation and helps muscles recover from pain. The best part is that it is able to burn calories easily, which enables you to lose as much fat as possible.

Ginger is also a great way to help regulate your blood sugar and leptin levels. Leptin, of course, is what helps you feel full after a meal and what keeps you from finding something else to eat right after you eat a meal. Ginger is also helpful when burning belly fat in particular. The main causes of belly fat are from overeating and lack of exercise. There is also a hormone that helps control the fat stored in the belly. For overeating, ginger helps you feel full. A good way to ensure that you don't overeat is by drinking some ginger water or just eating a little ginger.

It can also give you some energy, which will help you get the motivation to go out and get some exercise in. A lot of the time, it's a lack of energy that stops people from going and exercising. Blood cortisol, when it is elevated, can cause a change in metabolism and the immune system. This can be elevated when there is a lot of chronic stress or a hormonal imbalance. Ginger is a regulator for your blood cortisol level, which, in turn, regulates your metabolism. As long as you eat enough ginger, you won't have to worry about your blood cortisol levels messing your metabolism up in any way.

Avocado

Avocados are full of mono-saturated fats and are easily digested to release calcium in the body. This ensures that while losing weight, your body stays healthy and maintains strong bones. When the body absorbs calcium, fat burn is encouraged. This makes avocados extremely good for you. It also is a great way to lower your cholesterol. It specifically targets the bad cholesterol and stops it from doing what it does. With the monounsaturated fats, they have been shown to prevent the distribution of fat in the belly, so eating an avocado every day might be exactly what you need.

Soybeans

Aside from helping you lose weight, soybeans also promote muscle building to keep your body strong and healthy. They also decrease calorie intake and appetite. Soybeans are a wonderful addition to many meals that you'll make. They are also a great source of calcium, vitamin K, Vitamin B2, dietary fiber, omega-3 fatty acids, iron, and potassium. Not only will you be eating to lose some weight, but also getting the nutrients you need.

Salmon

Salmon is also rich in Omega-3 Fatty Acids. It can provide your body with most of the energy that it needs. This means that fat burning can easily occur and that your metabolism can increase. However, you'll want to be aware of how you cook it. Using things like butter to cook it will add to the fat content of it. Maybe try broiling the salmon instead, adding the herbs that you want. This way, you'll know for sure that you aren't making the dish more fattening than it needs to be. Without butter, it is a lean source of protein, which makes it a great food to eat that will keep you feeling full.

Of course, the fish oil that is in salmon also plays a big part in losing weight. Fish oil is where the Omega-3 Fatty Acids come from, so you know that you'll be losing some weight if you eat salmon. A great thing about salmon is that there is Vitamin D in them, something that is not often found in foods. Vitamin D is one of the harder vitamins to find in food, so you should take it where you can find it. The benefits of Vitamin D have already been talked about, so if you want to learn more, go back in the book and find it in the nutrient section.

Grapefruit

By eating grapefruit at least thrice a day, you will be able to lose around 4 pounds in 12 weeks, even without exercise! This is why this fruit is included in most diet plans. Grapefruit reduces the body's insulin levels. Insulin controls blood sugar levels and prevents fat from entering or being stored in the body.

Grapefruit is considered a superfood. It is very dense in nutrients, making it a wonderful food to snack on and eat. If you ever needed a food that has Vitamin C, you've found it. One interesting thing about grapefruit is that even smelling it has benefits. In fact, when you smell a grapefruit, specifically the oil, it slows down the nerve in your body that calls for the munchies. This means that you can go longer without eating, since your body doesn't think it needs to eat.

There are enzymes in grapefruit that help break down fats. This way, they won't get stored and add to your weight. Instead, they will be broken down and gotten rid of, making your road to weight loss much easier. Cellulite is something many people deal with on a daily basis. Fortunately, grapefruit has something in it that naturally gets rid of cellulite, making your skin look much smoother and nicer. Plus, if you need a good immune system boost, grapefruit might be where you need to go. Thanks to the huge amount of Vitamin C, you might be more easily able to fight off infections and illnesses thanks to grapefruit.

Flax Seeds

Flax seeds are also full of Omega-3 Fatty Acids that again lead to increased metabolic levels. Along with this, flax seeds are very high in fiber, which helps reduce your appetite by keeping you feeling full for longer. It is important to keep in mind that flax seeds are among the foods with the most amount of calories. How, then, do you burn away the calories that you gained through eating flax seeds? Exercise, of course, is the easiest thing to go with. This will ensure that you are definitely burning everything off and aren't leaving unwanted calories behind. Otherwise, if exercise isn't an option right now, you should look at other foods, like cauliflower. This is also high in fiber, but doesn't have nearly as many fat calories as flax seeds have.

Of course, you can always just have a smaller portion of the flax seeds if you are very worried about the amount of calories you'll be consuming. Just because something seems hard with calories doesn't mean you have to make it harder by not eating something you want to eat. Working out is the easiest way to get away with eating something like flax seeds and still having all the benefits that they bring.

Peanut Butter

Contrary to popular belief, peanut butter is not fattening. It's a great source of healthy fats. However, some manufacturers change ingredients, so always be sure to check nutrition labels.

The most effective way to have peanut butter be in your weight loss diet is mixing it with other foods. Fruit is a wonderful thing to mix your peanut butter with. It will make the snack healthier and give you a reason to eat peanut butter. Another thing to do is control your portion size of peanut butter. Believe it or not, but it doesn't take much peanut butter to be a serving. Therefore, you should figure out how much peanut butter is in one serving and using that much every time you eat it. You'll then know exactly how much you are eating rather than just taking it out of the jar and continuously eating it. Plus, a great thing about peanut butter and regular nuts is the decrease of the chances of heart disease.

Honey

Honey is a form of sugar, but it has a low glycemic index, which means that your metabolism levels continue to burn instead of store fat. It also helps fat cells release fat energy so that fat can be used and not stored in your body. In additions, honey is a great anti-oxidant!

One way to use honey is by using it in place of sugar. Since it still contains sugar, you can use it in a recipe that calls for sugar and not have to worry about it being just sugar. Honey actually contains a bunch of vitamins and minerals, making it a great thing to have with a snack. There are also a few combinations that are popular with honey, including honey and water, honey and lemon juice, and honey and cinnamon. Each of these have their own benefits for weight loss. Here is a brief breakdown of the benefits for all three.

Honey and warm water has been shown to mobilize stored fat. This makes it easier to burn when you go through your exercise routine. Also, since honey reduces the risk of stroke and heart attack, you won't have to worry about those when doing your exercises. All of this has been said to be stimulated by mixing honey and warm water.

Honey and lemon juice is mixed specifically for weight loss. The nutrients in honey, especially the amino acids, are perfect for stimulating the metabolism. You'll be able to see the weight slowly drop off as you drink this concoction. Lemon juice, on the other hand, is perfect for increasing your liver function and increasing your fat metabolism. Plus, this concoction is also perfect for going on a cleanse.

Honey, cinnamon, and warm water is another great combination. Cinnamon has been researched and people have found that it has some weight loss benefits. It has been shown to regulate blood sugar levels and regulate the metabolism of glucose. Both of these are very important when it comes to losing weight. Drinking this on an empty stomach is the recommended way to do it, as it will give the greatest effect on your body. Without question, this is a wonderful way to lose some weight naturally.

Broccoli

Broccoli is high in fiber and thus helps you maintain a low blood sugar level and keeps you feeling full longer. Broccoli is also one of the most concentrated sources of Vitamin C, which we already know is a powerful anti-oxidant. Broccoli, overall, is a great snack food. With the amount of nutrients in broccoli, you won't have to worry about finding an unhealthy snack to munch on. Instead, you can just have a few pieces of raw broccoli and eat that. The phytochemicals in broccoli are also attributed to weight loss. These are said to help with the breakdown of fat cells. You'll see some weight fall off as you eat more things like broccoli.

Chili Pepper Flakes

Chili pepper flakes contain capsaicin, an enzyme that comes from hot peppers that are included in chili pepper flakes, such as chili peppers, ancho, and cayenne. These peppers are good choices because the capsaicin that they contain increases metabolism to burn fat and suppress appetite. Adding these to a drink is a great way to start the day. Not only will it give your drink a little heat, but will also jumpstart your metabolism. Then, you can go through the day, not worrying as much about what you're eating. You can relax a little and instead focus on things that you need to do. Chili pepper flakes can also burn stored fat, making it even better.

Eggs

Eggs should be one of the mainstays of a healthy diet. Start your day by eating eggs, and you'll find you won't be looking for fatty foods throughout the day. Eggs are a great source of protein, which is essential in maintaining a healthy body and a well-balanced diet. It is great for feeding fussy kids. It can serve as a quick snack, lunch, or supper and as an ingredient for all kinds of culinary dishes.

For decades, the egg has been blamed for all sorts of health problems because of its high cholesterol content. For years, eggs were shunned, and people ate only the whites. The American Heart Association then reversed its guidelines and advised an egg per day. In one of the many studies that food scientists conduct, it was discovered that the high cholesterol in eggs is not associated with heart disease. Instead, heart disease was attributed to saturated fats, but even this advice is now in dispute (see Dairy). All the blame here should not be laid at the door of scientists. It is just that the whole subject of food and the effects it has on our body are so vast that the information we have is constantly evolving. This is all the more reason to stick to natural, unprocessed products whenever possible. After all, this is what our ancestors lived on for thousands of years.

Egg whites, of course, are the best part of the egg when looking only at weight loss. However, you do still need to realize that the yolk has a ton of vitamins that you will miss out on if you stick with only eating egg whites. Therefore, you should mix it up, having only egg whites some days and having the whole egg other days. The best thing about eggs is how filling they are. You won't feel yourself getting hungry an hour after eating eggs. Instead, you will feel more satisfied with the foods you're eating and not have to find a snack to munch on. You'll be less inclined on finding a cheap, fattening snack if you have eggs in the morning.

Plus, a great thing about eggs is that they are cheap and easy to prepare. They only take a few minutes in the morning to cook and are anything but difficult. There are different variations as well. You can scramble them, poach them, make and omelet, or do a bunch of other things. You can have eggs a different way every morning and add things to them, like bell pepper, spinach, and other healthy items. You can make different kinds of eggs every morning and never feel like you are eating the same thing. Plus, you'll know that what you're eating is healthy and only beneficial.

Olive Oil

The reason why olive oil is used in most diets is because it is extremely beneficial in terms of fat and calorie burning, given that it helps the body make use of fat as energy. It also improves cardiovascular health and aids the immune system in protecting you against viruses. It likewise keeps you safe from most heart ailments and lowers the risk of stroke.

Olive oil should be the first thing you turn to when you need a kind of oil. The benefits are much higher than other types of oils. Olive oil is made with monounsaturated fats, which is one of the good fats. This brings down the bad cholesterol and brings up the good cholesterol. It also decreases the chance of heart disease, which is always a big plus.

All of these foods can help you lose weight in some way. Many of them have similar nutrients, so make sure to look into what nutrients are most beneficial for weight loss so you can choose your foods accordingly, especially if you have any food allergies.

Chapter 6: Other Reminders

Here are a couple of reminders to you keep focused on eating the right kinds of food so that you lose weight safely and as quickly as possible while maintaining peak health.

Fat

Always choose lean meat over fatty meat, and go for grass-fed ones as often as possible.

Remember, you don't need to eliminate all fats from your diet. As mentioned earlier, there are good fats and bad fats. Just be sure to choose the right ones as often as possible. Go for polyunsaturated and monounsaturated fats before you go with saturated. These are the best fats for your heart and your overall health.

Protein

Cooking chicken or any other meat in shortening or margarine adds to the amount of fat intake, even if the meat is rich in protein. Always choose to cook your meats in olive oil instead.

Try to take off any skin on chicken or buy chicken that is skinless. The skin on chicken is easily the most fattening part, so avoid it if you can.

Processed meats, such as frankfurters, sausage, and ham, already have sodium because salt is used to help preserve them. This means that you should limit your intake of these foods and that you should always check their nutrition labels. Check for the words "self-basting" or "contains ___ % of sodium" to see how much sodium they contain.

Seafood rich in Omega-3 Fatty Acids are some of your best choices when it comes to protein-rich foods. These include sardines, salmon, trout, anchovies, Pacific oysters, and herring.

Unsalted nuts should be chosen over salted nuts each time. Also, try to have these unsalted nuts near you. They are a great snack food that will keep you going throughout the day. They are better than grabbing a bag of chips.

Grains

The modern diet includes huge amounts of grain. We eat it directly in such forms as rice, and we eat it indirectly when it is processed into everyday items, such as bread. We also find it as a frequently used product in other areas where we might not expect it at all when it is employed to bulk up processed food.

Grains are a good source of complex carbohydrates, as well as some key vitamins and minerals. The problem is that very often, the ingredients that are good for us are removed during the refining process, and we are left with a large amount of carbohydrates and little or nothing else. This becomes particularly bad when we over eat things such as cookies and pastries, where we receive virtually no goodness but only plenty of sugar.

To avoid falling into this trap, the best grains to go for are whole grains. Whole grains have not been milled, and as such, they still have the bran and germ. Bran and germ are the sources of most of the nutrients we are after and virtually all the fiber. Fiber is important because it fills us up and helps reduce appetite. We have acquired a taste for refined grains, such as white flour, and this is helpful to the food industry because such grains increase the shelf life of their products. At least half your grains should come in the form of whole grain products. Don't be fooled by non-whole-grain brown bread either. Having discovered that their client base was starting to move toward healthier brown bread, some manufacturers started adding colorants to white bread to give the impression that they were selling a healthier option. Check the nutrition panel, and make sure the word "whole" appears very high on the list. There is also a white whole grain that is perfectly healthy.

There are several ways to increase your daily intake of whole grains aside from just buying whole grain bread. Try replacing white rice with brown rice, kasha, wild rice, or crushed bulgur wheat. White rice has seventy-five percent less nutrients than brown rice, and it has less antioxidants, magnesium, phosphorus, and vitamin B. It is quite astonishing how simply changing from white to brown rice can improve your diet. and for an additional change, there is also red and black rice that are equally healthy.

Start your day off with a whole grain cereal, such as whole grain bran or oats.

Below is a list of some grains that could serve as a tasty and healthy alternative to what you may be used to.

Whole grain Barley

This is great in soups and stews. This can be beneficial in lowering glucose levels, something that is always helpful when trying to lose weight. If you add this to your diet every day, you'll notice a big change in your body. You might actually have more energy after eating this.

Whole Grain Rye

This contains four times more fiber and fifty percent more daily iron than any other whole grain. A great thing about this is that it helps you feel full much faster than other grains do. This is mostly due to the fiber, which sticks to water and absorbs it. For weight loss, whole grain rye might be the exact grain you want to go with.

Buckwheat

Actually a seed, it can be served like rice or made into porridge. This has a lot of benefits, including being very good for your cardiovascular health. It can also lower your risk of diabetes, since it lowers your blood sugar and helps regulate it. Magnesium is a big part of buckwheat, which is one of the reasons that it helps with blood sugar and diabetes. With that, it helps lower the blood glucose levels, making them much healthier and less likely to cause issues in the future.

Whole Wheat Couscous

This is very quick and easy to prepare and is an ideal white rice substitute. Couscous, especially whole wheat, is wonderful for improving your cardiovascular health. Selenium is a trace mineral in many different foods, but couscous has a good amount of it. Selenium is a mineral that is important to our health, so it's always good to find a food that has a lot of it. This is mainly a mineral that helps reduce plaque buildup in the arteries, especially around your heart. This is what leads to heart attacks. Therefore, eating plenty of couscous will lower the chances of having a heart attack.

Couscous is also a great thing to eat for cancer prevention. Selenium, once again, has been seen to reduce the chances of prostate cancer specifically, as a deficiency has been seen to increase the chances of that particular cancer. There are still studies going on to prove if selenium is good for other cancer prevention as well, but it is still ongoing. If you want to improve your muscle mass, then eating couscous will help. Selenium has also been linked to your muscle mass, including a deficiency making your muscles easier to degrade and harder to build up.

If you want an immune system boost, this food is also helpful with that. Selenium has been shown to stimulate the regeneration of Vitamin C and Vitamin E, which are both important for the immune system. Therefore, eating plenty of couscous could help your immune system be a lot stronger. Also, couscous can help with digestion. There is fiber in this, which has been proven to help with all sorts of things, including digestion. Overall, couscous is a wonderful food that has a ton of benefits.

Corn

Yes, whole corn is healthy and easy to eat in the form of popcorn, but you should avoid the microwave versions.

Quinoa

This is really a seed, but it contains four times more protein than any other grain. This is also high in Omega-3. Quinoa is a wonderful seed that can be used in a lot of different ways. It has so many nutrients in it and it makes a wonderful alternative to rice. It is a great side dish to add to any meal, but especially a meal with some sort of pork or steak. Quinoa also has things called flavonoids, which are natural plant antioxidants. The two big flavonoids in quinoa are quercetin and kaempferol. These have been shown to be anti-inflammatory, anti-cancer, anti-viral, and anti-depressant. All of these things are very important and are a great thing to have in a single food.

The amount of fiber in quinoa is also something to keep in mind. It has more fiber than a lot of other grains. In a way, quinoa could almost be considered a superfood in grains. Even though there is a lot of fiber, most of it isn't beneficial to your health. However, there is still a good amount of soluble fiber which is very beneficial. Therefore, even though there might not be as much as anyone would like, it's still a great food for fiber.

If gluten is an issue, here's a wonderful, gluten free grain. You won't have to worry about an intolerance with this, making it the perfect food for you to eat. One reason this food is known for its protein is because it contains all the essential amino acids. When a food does this, it is considered a complete protein. Therefore, quinoa is seen as a complete protein. It's pretty interesting to think about, especially since this is a grain, not a protein. Most people think of meat having all the protein, but they neglect to think about things like quinoa. You should always keep you mind open when it comes to foods and the nutrients that you need.

There are tons of antioxidants in this grain as well. All of this only makes it easier for you to see why this is such an important grain to keep in mind. There was a study done about the number of antioxidants in foods. Ten foods were studied and out of those ten, quinoa had the most.

Freekeh

This is an ancient wheat that can be eaten like rice. It contains four times the fiber of brown rice. This has often been compared to quinoa, which has become a favorite in the grain world. In many ways, it's better than quinoa. There are more nutrients in freekeh than in quinoa and more of those nutrients. One big thing that quinoa has over freekeh is the fact that freekeh is not gluten free. It is a wheat, after all. However, that doesn't make anything that freekeh has less relevant. There is a ton of fiber in freekeh, making it a great source of fiber. This means you'll feel fuller after eating, making you snack less frequently. Freekeh is easily a super grain to be looking out for.

Some products include bran, which is a good source of fiber. However, you need to consider that if bran has been added, such as oat bran, this is not a whole grain product.

There are also some grains that are made from a mixture of refined and whole grains, so as a reminder, be sure to check nutrition labels.

Dairy

When I was a kid, we were given a small bottle of full cream milk every day at school. It was also the go-to drink for healthy kids, way before pop and fizzy drinks became the norm. Fizzy drinks were restricted to parties and other treats. Then came the low-fat revolution, and we were told to avoid any dairy that was not low-fat or skimmed so that we can reduce our intake of saturated fats, which we were told caused of so many health problems in the western diet. Now, the scientific world is divided over whether this advice was correct or not. The European Journal of Nutrition has produced a study that says that people who eat full fat dairy are no more likely to develop cardiovascular disease or type 2 diabetes than those on low fat. Moreover, the study claims that in terms of weight gain, full cream may be better for you. Remember that we mentioned the appestat, which helps you determine when you have had enough in terms of fat.

That single scientific study may have been an off-the-wall work that we should disregard, except that more and more studies are coming through that support its findings. Moreover, health authorities who have been caught on the back foot are having to rethink their advice. I don't want to get into a debate that is still raging in the scientific world other than to say that the more natural a product is and the less it has been tampered with by the food industry, the more I trust it.

If you are not ready to abandon the low-fat and skimmed options that now line the supermarket shelves, that is okay, but don't abandon dairy altogether unless you are dairy intolerant. Dairy is a great source of protein, calcium, magnesium, as well as vitamins A, D, and E, so you need to include it in a healthy diet. Dairy is a very important thing, especially for children who are still developing. Milk is especially important, as it contains a lot of minerals and vitamins. One of the proteins found in milk is a complete protein, with all the essential amino acids in it. The antibodies that protein helps create are extremely important in children who are growing. They need to have the easiest time fighting off infections, since children tend to be more vulnerable to a lot of illnesses. Therefore, the more antibodies they have, the stronger their immune system is. No one likes seeing their child sick, so make sure they drink milk.

Of course, that doesn't make milk and other dairy products any less important for adults. Like I stated earlier, milk has tons of vitamins and minerals. These are just as essential for adults as they are for children. They are even more important in some cases. Calcium is especially important for people who are aging. You don't want to develop something like osteoporosis, which is the degradation of your bones. Instead, you should aim to continue strengthening them as much as possible. Milk can be a great way to get the extra calcium that you need.

Other dairy products are also just as important. Always make sure to look at the nutrition labels to find out exactly what is in each of the dairy products, especially with cheese. Some cheeses have more fat than others, so you'll want to be aware of which ones are healthier.

There are tons of different foods out there. These are some of the essentials that you should keep in mind. Always look for the healthiest things that you can when it comes to foods. The healthier, the better. In fact, if you have something that falls into one of these categories every day, you might find yourself going for the healthier options every day rather than just when you think about it. Every time you go shopping, looking for another item to add to your weekly food that's healthy. Soon, you'll notice that everything in your cart is healthy and you'll know that you're making the right choice.

Chapter 7: Getting Started

All of the above chapters may be a little intimidating and confusing, so the best thing to do is just look at how to get started and how to keep things as simple as possible. First, you need to know what it is that you want to achieve. Remember that even if you are not carrying excess weight, your body is simply not performing as well as it could if you are not eating a healthy balanced diet, and over the long term, there might be health implications.

Being Mindful Of What We Eat

We have become conditioned by a number of factors when we eat. The large food companies have molded many of our eating habits, but they are not alone in taking responsibility for the health of our nations. We also have to change well-established habits and addictions and though it may seem counter intuitive, this often starts with the mind. In many cases, we have become emotional eaters who allow our mood or circumstances to dictate what we consume rather than taking a few minutes to think things through and opt for the healthiest choices. With the information above, we are now able to make informed decisions, but we probably already knew some of that information. However, we still failed to act on it. Much of this boils down to time. We grab meals on the run, multi-task whilst eating, and sometimes, don't even sit down to appreciate our meal. Worse is that we are in such a hurry that we fail to listen to our body when it says it is full, and instead, we gorge ourselves.

There are even times where we are sitting at home and absentmindedly grab a snack that we know that we shouldn't eat. Maybe there's some chips laying around that you snack on while watching your favorite TV show. Maybe you have some candy that's sitting in a bowl on your living room table. Then, you just go and grab it without thinking, just eating it. This is definitely not helpful if you are trying to change your lifestyle.

Here are a few tips that might help you to not only eat less, but also enjoy your food more.

Start with the purchase. Make a list in advance, and have an idea what you are shopping for rather than just throwing things into your basket when you are at the supermarket or store. I find that it is a bad idea to shop on an empty stomach as I tend to do more impulse buying. Think about each item before placing it in the basket, and take the time to read the nutrition charts if you are not sure of what each item contains. With each item, think about the impact it will this have on your health.

Once you get home with your groceries, decide on the best way to prepare them, and then enjoy the cooking process. Further on in the book, I will share a few easy-to-prepare yet healthy meals to get you started. Although there are thousands of healthy eating cookery books out there to add to the recipes I will provide, always aim for quality over quantity.

If realistic, sit down at the table with your healthily prepared meal after switching of the television and internet. Now enjoy your meal and give it the respect it deserves by eating it slowly. Put your cutlery down between mouthfuls, and chew slowly and deliberately. This will not only let you enjoy your food more, but it will also aid in your digestion.

Stop eating when you feel full. Aim to be slightly hungry when you reach the end of your meal, and then stop eating. Wait for twenty minutes, and then reassess to see if you are still hungry. It takes a while for the stomach to get the right signals up to the brain so that it knows you are full. Once you have done this for a few days, you will be amazed at how much less you eat.

Always have a jug of water on the table, and make sure you drink a glass or two during the course of your meal. This slows down that speed at which you eat, helps you feel full earlier, and aids digestion.

Feel free to leave food on your plate when you are full. If you grew up in a home like mine, you were probably often encouraged to eat everything placed in front of you, regardless of whether you were full on not Because of something about the poor starving children in Africa or Asia. How that little lesson has damaged our eating habits! Instead of trying to force down every morsel on the plate, ask yourself, "Do I really want this?" If the answer is no, then leave it. It certainly does not need to go to waste. We live in the age of refrigerators, and leftovers can be made delicious. Would you rather that it be in the refrigerator or stored on your hips as fat your body could not process?

I know that this sounds impossibly unrealistic in terms of time, but what price is your health worth, and how much time will you lose if you have some major health problem develop as a result of hastily thought out, badly prepared, and gulped down meals? There was a time when we had a love affair with food. It played a major role in every reunion, from christenings to funerals, from weddings to birthdays. Over the past decade, we have seen a huge increase in the number of cooking programs, and many of these programs are very popular. The problem is that there doesn't seem to be a relationship between what people watch on their television and what they do in their kitchens. All over the world, people are sitting down to watch a healthy cooking program whilst munching on fast food. How crazy is that?

We need to rebuild that love affair again and stop poisoning our bodies with food that somebody else has prepared with no consideration for anything other than how cheaply it can be made and how they can increase their profits.

Don't Beat Yourself Up

The road to healthy eating is a long, slow one. Think of it as a marathon rather than a sprint. Along the way, there will be days that you may fall off the wagon. There will be dinner parties, company get-togethers, or just plain pig outs where you find yourself shoving jam doughnuts into your mouth. It happens. You haven't failed, and your body is a pretty robust machine. It will forgive you. You must learn to forgive yourself, put it behind you, and go straight back into your health routine. It is all too easy to say, "Okay, I've failed for a day. What is the point in carrying on?"

It's easy to give up. It's much harder to accept that it didn't go exactly how you wanted, but you still move on and keep going. Let yourself have some moments where you think of all the good that is coming from changing your eating habits. If your goal is losing weight, keep a weekly tab of the foods you ate and your weight. It's okay if it isn't exactly where you want it. Everything to do with this is a process, so allow it to be what it is. Don't try to force something to happen when it shouldn't. Everything will come in time.

If you need to, schedule a specific cheat day. Set ground rules for that cheat day. Do everything in your power to give yourself the power to succeed. You can easily set yourself up to fail, but you can just as easily set yourself up to succeed. If you like a lot of structure, give yourself structure within your diet. If you need a little wiggle room, give it to yourself. You need to realize that everything with your diet is in your own hands. Someone else isn't making these choices for you, it's all on you. Tell yourself you can do it and you'll be surprised at what you can accomplish.

Chapter 8: Some Tips On Shopping And Recipes

Naturally, how we shop is going to affect how we eat. If you can restrict yourself to eating when you get home rather than buying fast food when you are on your way home, then you have much greater control of how healthy your food is going to be. Of course, this is going to break down if you go home to an empty refrigerator or when what you have in the refrigerator is unhealthy. I know there are going to be days when you arrive home and cannot summon up the energy to cook a full meal. Later, we will look at some tips for having healthy standbys that can be just popped into the microwave for a few minutes. For now though, we will look at what items you should have in the fridge, freezer, and cupboards.

As previously mentioned, it is important to have a shopping list before you go. If you have already drawn up a weekly meal plan, then having to make a list should not be too difficult. Remember to try not to shopping when you are hungry. There are several studies that show that shopping whilst hungry leads to increased spending and not always on the right things. Many times, going to the store hungry results in quick and easy foods. You're already hungry, so why would you want to spend an hour cooking something when you can just put it in the microwave for a few minutes?

A great tip is to plan out what you want to make throughout the week. Do you have your heart set on having a steak at some point this week? Write it down when you have the thought. Every time you think of something you want to make for dinner in the next week, be sure to write it down. There have been plenty of times that I've gone to the store with a few things in mind and realized a few days later that it was not enough food. Always make sure that you get enough food for the entire week. Planning ahead is a good idea not only so you know that you have enough food, but if you end up making something else one night, you'll still have what you didn't make ready to go.

If you can, going to a store where you can buy food in bulk is always a great option. Maybe you know that you are going to have a bunch of people over for a get together. You can buy the things you need in bulk instead of spending more money and getting the same amount at a different store. Things like juice are great when bought in bulk, especially if you and your family drinks a lot of juice. You won't have to worry about running out of it in the middle of the week and needing to buy more.

Meat and fish are going to be the most expensive items on most people's shopping list. There are several options here to make your money go further while eating more cheaply. First, look for cheaper cuts. Chicken thighs, for example, are normally cheaper than chicken breasts. Cheaper still is buying whole chicken and then roasting it. This will give you a great first meal with leftovers that can be used for more meals later. There are many recipes, such as stew and casseroles, which combine meat and vegetables to make the meat go further. These options will allow you to use slightly cheaper meat cuts, such as stewing steak. Also, make sure to try to buy chicken that is skinless. This will help with your fat intake. If the skinless is more expensive, buy the skinned chicken and take it off before you start cooking. Either way, you will be getting a food that is much healthier and less fattening while still getting the best bang for your buck. Buying frozen or canned fish is often the cheapest way to go, and there is nothing unhealthy about these options. Some of the cheapest frozen fish can be quite bland, but cooked when with a nice sauce, the frozen fish soon turns into a delicious healthy meal at a much cheaper price than fresh fish. There are plenty of people who live a vegetarian lifestyle, and for them, the meat buying problem falls out of the equation. I am no vegetarian, but I do recognize that we eat too much meat and that large-scale meat production negatively affects the environment. I am not ready to let go of my steak lust just yet, but I do observe meat-free Mondays that has become a huge movement. By giving up meat one day a week (it doesn't need to be a Monday), we can help the environment and our shopping at the same time.

Meats are obviously incredibly important to any diet, as long as you still eat meat. Take your time to look at the various meats available wherever you are getting your groceries from. Make sure they look the way you want and are lean. Don't cart the first one you see, but take time to look. You might be surprised at how much better tasting the meat is that you find.

Pulses are both cheap and healthy. and they are a great addition to meat dishes, or they can replace meats from time to time.

I am not going to tell you not to go to the supermarket to do your shopping. For convenience, supermarkets are hard to beat, but they are not always the best option, especially when buying fresh vegetables. Vegetables are the mainstay of a healthy diet, but supermarkets often import them from distant countries. This affects both their nutrition levels and price. Try to buy vegetables that are in season and grown locally. Often, there will be sales on items that they suddenly find they have a glut of. This is the time to buy these food items and then pop them in the freezer. Corn, for example, will cost a fortune in the non-summer months, but the price goes through the floor in summer, so buy loads and throw it in the freezer then.

If you have the land and knowledge, you should grow your own vegetables. With a big enough garden, you'll be able to grow tons of vegetables that can then be frozen and used later. This does take some time to do and not everyone has the kind of time that it takes, but at least you will know exactly where the food is coming from. You'll know that it's healthy and definitely not drenched in preservatives or chemicals. Fruit trees are also a great idea, if you have the space for them. Any way that you can save on buying healthy fruits and vegetables should be taken.

Pre-frozen vegetables are almost always cheaper. They are convenient and will have been frozen shortly after picking, so they lose very little of their nutrition levels. Even canned vegetables are both nutritious and convenient, but be sure to check the nutrition chart to see what additives, especially sugar and salt, may have been placed into the can.

If you have a farmer's market nearby, this is one of the best sources of high-quality fruit and vegetables. If you are in an area where you know some of the farmers, then you might be buying from people that you know. You'll be more inclined to buy from them if it's someone that you know. Moreover, you are supporting an industry that is coming under lots of pressure. Towards the end of the day, they will often sell off stock more cheaply to avoid having to pack it up and take it back to the farm with them. Wherever you buy your vegetables, remember to go for a rainbow of colors to get plenty of variety.

If you have the space, then it pays to buy healthy foods in bulk. Aside from helps on price, you are virtually assured that you will always be able to find something healthy to eat in your kitchen, and that is a good way to avoid eating junk. I always have tubs of yoghurt, fruit, and almonds in the house. No matter what happens, I know I can combine those three ingredients to have a healthy snack or meal if ever I need one.

Because I try to buy less, I prefer to go for the smallest shopping trolley I can find. Another useful tip is to shop when the supermarket is not full, if possible. Supermarkets are designed so that there are plenty of impulse choices in view while you stand in queue, and this is a sure way to find things you don't need sneaking into the trolley. In fact, you should stick with your list and nothing else. Pretend that the rest of the store isn't even there. All that's there are the groceries you need and the list that you made. Go straight to those items and put them in your cart before you can look at something else. Obviously, with things like fruit, vegetables, and meats, look only at the things that you want to buy to make sure you buy the best ones possible. However, don't let your eyes wander to other things that surround the things on your list. Any way to avoid an impulse buy is important.

Cutting Down Food Waste

As much as forty percent of food produced in America gets thrown away. The figures for Europe and Britain are not much better. That waste does not all happen in our kitchens, as plenty is wasted on the farm and during the transport and manufacturing processes, but there is still a huge amount of domestic food waste taking place. Much of that will start to decrease automatically as you start becoming more conscious of what you buy and start buying what you need rather than what you think you want on impulse. Here are a few tips to reduce food waste further.

One good place to reduce waste is the refrigerator. Keeping it organized helps reduce waste in that you can eat the oldest food first, and you can be sure that there are no items tucked away that you have forgotten about. Placing in cold water for a few minutes can revive greens that look sad and wilted. Scraps can be turned into snacks or meals and added to other dishes.

When you buy in bulk, be sure to store the oldest items at the front of your cupboards, and put the newer ones behind them.

Many recipes will list a specific ingredient that you don't have. Try replacing it with another similar ingredient that you do have. If something needs a milk based product that you don't have, you can try to replace it with milk. This way, you'll be able to still make what you want without any issue.

Have some good airtight containers for storing items like nuts for longer. Also, keep them in a space that you will see, especially if they don't need to be refrigerated. This will ensure that they will get eaten by someone, since they are in an appetizing spot.

Have one meal a week that can be considered a use-it-up meal by putting together an assortment of leftovers that have accumulated in the refrigerator. Bread is one of the most frequently wasted items. Bread freezes really easily, especially if you halve the loaf and pop one half into the freezer before you even start to use it. If you tend to go through a lot of bread, it's easiest to buy a few loaves and put the extras in the freezer. That way, when you go through the first loaf, you can bring the next one out without needing to go back to the store to get another one. Of course, if you aren't a frequent bread eater, buying bread that is a smaller loaf might be the best idea for you. There are some breads which come in smaller loafs, making it easier for you.

Often, people forget about the foods that they have in their kitchen. If you can, put foods that you don't want to forget about in places where you will definitely see them. Don't put something like salmon on the counter, of course, but if you have some oatmeal that you keep forgetting about, put it on the counter so you'll see it right when you walk into the kitchen in the morning. Doing this is even more important when you buy in bulk. Buying in bulk is good, but not if you buy too much of something that will go bad. Keep those things in places that you will always see to ensure that they will be eaten.

Finally, learn to monitor what you throw away so that you start to get a handle on your greatest areas of waste, and then alter you shopping accordingly. If you tend to throw away fruit every week, maybe it's time to stop buying that fruit. Maybe there's a certain meal you make too much of every time and the leftovers never get eaten. Try making a smaller batch of that food next time so that it is eaten when you make it. Then, you won't have to worry about leftovers.

Putting It Into Practice

Below are some simple recipes followed by a meal plan that will help you get started on your new healthy lifestyle program. This is by no means a comprehensive collection, but it will certainly give you some ideas both on how to eat and what to shop for. After that, you can start to introduce your own innovations based on the information you now have. You can also start to gather other healthy recipes. There are plenty of recipes available to you through the internet and through cookbooks. If you ever want to find more, they aren't hard to find. Remember that food is your friend, and you have to start to develop a different relationship with the food you put into your body while eliminating the careless attitude of the past. By giving a little thought, a little time, and a little patience, you will find yourself feeling and looking better.

It will likely be hard at first. It might seem like there's no way it will ever work out in your favor. If you can, try to start this with someone else. You can lean on each other when it starts to get hard and support each other when you are having issues. Plus, it's always more fun when you have someone else to do something like this with. Working together to do something generally means that it will happen in the end. If you can't do it with anyone else, if they don't want to or they can't for other reasons, that doesn't mean you won't be able to do it yourself. You need to know that you can do it yourself. It will be a little harder, but if you set yourself goals and see them through to the end, you will be much more successful than you would be otherwise. You might even surprise yourself with the great things you can do. Always tell yourself you have what it takes and great things will come your way. This is not a quick weight loss plan. It is a new, healthy, and sustainable lifestyle.

Breakfast Recipes

For years, breakfast has been promoted as the most important meal of the day. Science is now starting to show that is not quite as important as we were led to believe and that equal attention should be paid to the other meals of the day. However, breakfast still sets us up for the day ahead. The problem with breakfast is that very often, we neglect it as we dash about getting dressed, sorting out the kids for their day, and preparing for the combat of our commute to work. This is a time when we might not do too much mindful eating and instead be tempted to grab something unhealthy. It helps if you can prepare these meals the night before, but in the real world that we live in, this might be wishful thinking. Breakfast should be an exciting meal that helps wake you up and give you the energy you need to get through the first half of the day. Many people feel that not eating breakfast is better for weight loss. This isn't true. Skipping a meal just makes you hungrier by the time it's lunch, so you are more than likely going to eat a lot more than you actually need. Plus, your body won't have the energy it needs to get through the morning. You'll feel more tired and the things you need to do, like work, might seem even more annoying than they would if you had a full stomach. The recipes below are chosen for their simplicity and their ease of preparation:

A Real Quickie:

Quarter one apple

Cube 8 grams of cheese

¼ cup of almonds or walnuts

This is my go-to meal when I find myself pressed for time. I can pop it all into a zip lock bag and munch on it on the way to work. It also doubles as a handy snack when I find myself hungry between meals.

Ricotta Kick Off:

This comprises of three tablespoons of low fat ricotta spread over two slices of whole wheat bread. Top this with some sliced tomato and a few cubes of yellow pepper. Sprinkle lightly with crushed black pepper. This will give you some great protein to start the day off with plus a great tasting sandwich.

Fruit Shake:

Fruit shakes or smoothies are easy to make and great to drink at any time of day, but their easy preparation makes them ideal for breakfast. There is no limit to what you can throw into them, but my usual method is to throw one cup of milk, half a tub of plain yoghurt, and eight grams of almonds into a blender. To this, I add a bit of whatever fruit I happen to have handy. Berries like strawberries, raspberries, black currants, and blueberries are high in anti-oxidants while also adding flavor. For fruits with less flavor, I throw in one teaspoon of honey. A quick word of warning here—some blenders cannot cope with whole nuts, which may need to be chopped on a cutting board first.

Easy Oats:

Most people make rolled oats into porridge, which makes up a very healthy meal, but I prefer to eat my oats raw. Take three quarters of a cup of rolled oats. Pour on enough milk to soak them. Some people prefer to eat this meal quite dry, but I tend to let the oats soak well. Add some chopped nuts or blueberries, and then add a half teaspoon of honey if you find this all too bland. I can prepare this breakfast in a about a minute, and it simply doesn't get much healthier. Oats are great for lowering cholesterol, and they fill you up for a long time, so this little starter should easily carry you through to lunchtime.

Bran Waffle:

Toast a bran waffle, then coat it generously with a tablespoon of peanut butter. To add a bit more interest, add a sprinkle of sesame seeds or dried raisins. You can replace the waffle with whole grain bread or a bran muffin.

Sunday Special:

Once in a while, why not blast off your day with a bigger meal that you may prefer to treat as brunch? Grill two rashers of back bacon. In a pan lightly oiled with olive or coconut oil, fry a large sliced tomato and a cup full of fresh mushrooms, then fry or scramble two farm eggs. This meal should keep you going for hours. Mushrooms are one of the more filling vegetables, and tomatoes actually become healthier when heated because some of the nutrients are made more accessible to our bodies.

Easy Work Lunches

Lunch when working is another meal that we may find hard to really think about. This exposes us to the temptation of hitting that button on the vending machine. The meals below are low in calories and very easy to prepare and eat. They do not take long to make but it may be easiest to prepare them the night before. I know you are tired and don't want to be bothered. Focus on the person you want to be in terms of health and weight. Pretty soon, you will find yourself becoming accustomed to spending a few minutes each evening getting lunch ready for the next day at work. As time progresses, you will find that you have more energy as your body adapts to its new healthier regime. Lunch is especially important if you work somewhere for long hours. You need something to help get you through the day and help you feel happier throughout the day. The more times you eat lunch, the more you will notice that you can get through your work day in a better mood.

Turkey Wrap:

1 whole wheat wrap

3 slices of turkey

2 Tablespoons of humus

1 tablespoon of cream cottage cheese or goats cheese

1 hand full of baby spinach

Throwing all this together and wrapping it up really takes no time at all. You will probably spend more time looking for a lunch box than you will making this meal, and turkey is both cheap and low fat.

Black Bean Burrito:

1 whole wheat wrap

¼ of a cup of black beans (canned beans are fine)

½ a sliced avocado

¼ of a small red onion

1 teaspoon of sweet chili sauce

When I am making this meal, I tend to make two or three at a time and pop the others into the refrigerator.

Grilled Chicken And Cheese Sandwich:

2 slices of whole grain bread

½ a chicken breast

1 slice of Gouda cheese (any cheese will do)

2 table spoons of Greek yoghurt

3 slices of tomato

Lettuce (or rocket if I can get it)

If you have a refrigerator at work, you can store the ingredients there and make this up at work in less time than it would take you to get that chocolate bar out of the vending machine, which will probably swallow your money half the time anyway. The only problem is that pretty soon, everyone in the office would want what you've got.

Egg Tomato And Avocado Sandwich:

1 whole wheat muffin

1 large egg

1 tea spoon of olive oil

Half an avocado

Two slices of tomato

Okay, I admit we are stretching you here. You need to muster all your willpower and fry an egg. You also need to cut the muffin in half before loading in the ingredients. One handy little reminder here—don't leave the egg too soft. It won't travel well, and it would look bad running down the front of your top during that first meeting after lunch.

Quinoa Tabbouleh:

Salads are a great meal for work because not only are they are easy to make and healthy, but they also allow you to just make up the recipe according to what you have in the kitchen. You cannot ruin a salad, but be sure to include enough protein or fat to get you through the second half of your workday. Leaves and tomato are great, but you need something a little more substantial. The idea is to feel healthy, and it won't do if you are starving.

100 grams of Quinoa (cook it according to the instructions on the bag)

75 grams of parsley chopped finely

4 diced tomatoes

100 grams of cucumber diced

1 table spoon of olive oil

2 tablespoons of balsamic vinegar

Juice and zest of ½ a lemon

1 teaspoon of honey

¼ clove of crushed garlic

50 grams of rocket or lettuce

Small pinch of salt

Mix the olive oil, vinegar, lemon juice, honey, salt, and garlic to make your dressing. Finally, mix the other ingredients, and pour the dressing over the top.

Dinner

I am using the term dinner here on the assumption that you are a working person who may be having your main meal in the evening. Of course, these meals are interchangeable, so if you have a bit more time during the day, you may choose to make these your lunchtime meals. These are only suggestions to get you started and, hopefully, gently seduce you into a passion for cooking, which is essential to really healthy eating. Dinner is a pretty crucial meal time for people who work. There will likely be days where you miss out on lunch because you had too much work to do. Fortunately, dinner can still be a great time to pick up on any nutrients you missed out on the day. You can always have a very healthy dinner and pick yourself up from the long day you just had.

Chicken, Broccoli, And Brussels Sprout Salad:

2 skinned chicken breasts.

½ teaspoon of salt

2 broccoli stems

2 tablespoons olive oil

Juice of ½ a lemon

Ground black pepper

3 cups Brussels sprouts (finely sliced)

2 celery stalks

¼ Cup fresh parsley

4 grams Parmesan cheese

Place the chicken in a small pan, cover it with water, and add half of the salt. Bring the water to boil, then remove the pan from the heat and let it stand for fifteen minutes. Drain and rinse with cold water, then allow it to cool completely. When cool, shred into bite-sized pieces.

Peel the broccoli stem and then slice it into thin strips. In a large bowl, mix the olive oil, lemon juice, salt, and pepper. Finally, add the chicken, the strips of broccoli, the Brussels sprouts, nuts, and parsley, and mix all ingredients gently. You have just made a healthy meal for two.

Beef Chow Mein:

This is a very popular dish that you will find on nearly any Chinese menu, but perhaps not cooked with quite the same attention to health as this recipe below.

450 grams egg noodles

4 tablespoons of peanut or walnut oil

450 grams of lean beefsteak cut into strips

2 garlic clove crushed

1 teaspoon grated root ginger

1 green pepper thinly sliced

1 carrot thinly slice

2 celery sticks sliced

8 spring onions

1 tablespoon dry sherry

1 teaspoon Demerara sugar (dark brown sugar will do)

2 tablespoons soy sauce

A few drops of chili sauce or some chili flakes

Cook the noodles for four and a half minutes in boiling water, then drain and rinse under cold water. Toss the noodles in one tablespoon of peanut or walnut oil. Heat the remaining oil in a pre-heated wok, and then stir fry the beef for 3 to 4 minutes. Add the garlic and grated ginger, and stir fry for a further 30 seconds. Add the pepper, carrot, celery, and onions, and stir fry for 2 more minutes. Pour in the sugar, sherry soy sauce, and chili, and continue mixing for another minute.

Finally, stir in the noodles, and keep mixing until the whole mixture is warmed through. This meal serves four.

Beef And Peppers With Lemon Grass:

500 grams lean beef fillet

2 tablespoons vegetable oil

1 garlic clove chopped finely

1 lemon grass stalk finely shredded

Thumb-sized root ginger finely chopped

I red pepper thickly sliced

1 green pepper thickly sliced

1 onion thickly sliced

2 tablespoons lime juice

Salt and pepper

Serve with freshly cooked noodles or rice

Cut the beef into long strips. Heat the oil in a pre-heated wok to high heat. Add the beef, and stir fry for three minutes. Add the garlic, lemon grass, and the ginger, and then remove the wok from the heat. Remove the ingredients from the wok and set aside. Add the pepper and onions to the wok, and fry until the onion starts to become golden. Return the beef to the wok, and add the lime juice. Season the dish with salt and pepper. Serve with rice or noodles. This dish is meant for four people.

Ratatouille:

This recipe is one of my favorites because of sheer convenience and its abundance of vegetables. A large quantity can be made, and this can be eaten hot or cold or as an accompaniment to steak, chicken, or other protein. Cracking an egg over it makes for an easy meal to throw together at the last minute. Finally, it freezes really well, so a large quantity can be divided into several meals, each of which can be defrosted on occasions when time is in short supply.

2 large onions

6 cloves garlic (peeled and chopped)

3 courgettes (Zucchini)

2 red pepper (Capsicum)

1 kg aubergines (Egg plant)

1 kg peeled tomatoes. (Canned are fine)

150 grams black olives (Preferably without pips)

½ teaspoon of thyme

30 grams capers

Salt and pepper to season

2 tablespoons of olive oil

Lightly brown the onions. After three minutes, add the tomato, onion, garlic, thyme, and seasoning. Cook gently for a further 30 minutes, and while that is happening, dice the remaining vegetables into cubes. Warm the oil in a large pan or wok, and fry the peppers and the eggplant until soft and golden. Drain off the excess oil by laying the ingredients on a piece of kitchen paper. Now fry the zucchini until soft, and add all the ingredients, including the olives and simmer for a further half an hour. This recipe will give six helpings, so you can freeze anything you do not use, or you can double the quantities and make a really large batch and have several meals on standby for when you need them.

Desserts

If this healthy eating method is to be both viable and sustainable, then it needs to include some of the pleasures in life, such as desert. You might need to steer clear of the Black Forest chocolate cake or the banana toffee pudding, but there are still plenty of healthy options. I have already looked at smoothies and yoghurt with fruit nuts and honey, but what about a couple of more interesting recipes to make healthy eating that little bit more enjoyable? Dessert is one of those things that people never want to say no to. Even when you've had a large dinner, there's still a part of you that wants to have something sweet after your savory dinner. Thankfully, there are plenty of desserts out there that aren't as high with sugar content and can actually be beneficial to your health instead. Making your own desserts is a great way to ensure you're getting everything you need.

Red Fruit Brûlés:

This is a healthy version of the traditional Crème Brûlée. It is low in calories and only takes 10 minutes to cook. It is a great dessert for when you have guests.

450 gm / 1 lb. assorted red fruits such as red currents, black currents, cherries and strawberries (These can be bought frozen and defrosted)

150 ml / 5 fluid oz. Sour cream

150 ml / 5 fluid oz. Natural fromage frais

1 teaspoon vanilla essence

4 tablespoons Demerara sugar

Start by pre-heating the grill, and divide the red fruits equally between the four heat-proof ramekin dishes. Combine and mix fromage frais and sour cream, then stir in the vanilla essence. Gently spoon the mixture over the fruit trying, to cover the fruit as evenly as possible. Sprinkle 1 tablespoon of Demerara sugar over each of the bowls, then place under the hot grill until the sugar completely melts and begins to caramelize, which normally takes two to three mins. Allow to cool slightly before serving.

Mixed Fruit Crumble:

This easy-to-cook dessert can provide up to 12 helpings and is thus ideal for dinner parties or for several family meals. It works equally well with fresh or frozen fruit, and it doesn't need to be defrosted before cooking.

2 kg of mixed fruit – peeled, cored, and quartered apples and pears, blackberries, plums, and figs (feel free to change these ingredients according to what you have available)

Cinnamon

100 gm almond meal

100 gm desiccated coconut

50 gm plain flour

50 gm sugar

50 gm butter

1 tablespoon honey

Pre-heat oven to 180 degrees C.

Place the fruit in a large oven-proof serving dish, drizzle the honey over the fruit, and then sprinkle in the cinnamon. In another bowl, mix the flour, almond meal, coconut, sugar, and butter with your fingertips to form a crumbly texture. Gently sprinkle the crumbly mixture over the dish of fruit, covering it evenly.

Place in the pre-heated oven for 30 minutes or until the crust is golden brown.

Serve with a dollop of yogurt.

The Sensitive Subject Of Snacks

It is probably best if we deal with this subject head on because almost everyone reading this book is going to snack at some stage. This is particularly true when you first start to change your eating habits from the fast food guzzling you may have done in the past. At first, when you start to eat a healthier diet, your body will tell you it is starving simply because it is used to all the fat, salt, and sugar that you have been giving it before you changed your ways. As your body comes to realize that it is not in fact being treated so badly after all, these feelings will subside, but there are going to be times when snacks between meals become a necessity.

There is a myth that eating more frequently speeds up metabolism and that by doing so, you can actually lose weight. In fact, it has been proven that the more often we eat, the more calories we consume overall. Ideally, we would not need to eat between meals because we should consume the right amount at each meal to last us until the next one. This is not an ideal world, so we might as well make the best of it. The scientific name for snacking is Between Meal Eating Episodes or BMEE, and it has been widely practiced throughout our history. What has changed is the quality of the food we choose to snack on.

The first thing to recognize is that feeling hungry does not mean you have an emergency on your hands and thus need to respond immediately. Think about how hungry you really are, and decide on whether you really have to eat immediately. If, after a few moments reflection, you feel you can hold out until the next meal, then do so. On the other hand, if you are gritting your teeth in discomfort, then a snack may be the answer. The question is, of course, which snack to go for. You now know that fresh vegetables and fruit provide fiber and fill you up, so these are obvious choices to go for. If necessary, try having something healthy with them, such as guacamole, humus, or even a little peanut butter. Whichever choice you decide on, try to eat slowly, drink water, and think about what you are eating. One good rule of thumb is that your snack should not have more than one hundred calories.

Snacks don't have to be evil things that you steer clear of. Instead, they should be seen as something that can help you get through your day and not make you worry about your next meal when you should be working. Always keep in mind that snacking might be exactly what your body needs, especially if you accidently miss a meal.

Here are a few easy-to-eat snacks and the amount of calories they contain on average so that you can make more informed choices about what snacks to have.

Apple (medium) 95 calories

Red pepper 37 calories

Peach 58 calories

Orange 65 calories

20 Cherry tomatoes 61 calories

These are just a few examples, but they will give you an idea of how many calories there are in these items and how handy they are as a quick snack that won't blow your daily intake sky high. Another good snack that I find very useful is almonds, which have an average of one hundred calories for every thirteen nuts. They are easy to carry, make you feel full quickly, and have been proven to decrease the risk of heart disease. If you prepare in advance for the possibility of needing a snack, then you can make sure you are always prepared by having some nuts or an apple with you instead of just grabbing the first edible thing that comes along, which in this day and age is probably going to be some form of fast food.

For a slightly more complicated snack, but one that is both delicious and filling, why not try the cocoa power ball?

Cocoa Power Ball:

330 grams almond meal

½ teaspoon ground cinnamon

60 grams vanilla protein powder or powdered milk

2 tablespoons cocoa powder

16 fresh dates (pitted)

1 tablespoon vanilla extract

Some desiccated coconut to assist rolling

Place all ingredients, except the dates and the vanilla extract, into a food blender, and give them a quick whiz.

Chop the dates by hand, and add them and the vanilla to the mix in the food blender. Whiz the ingredients again until a sticky consistency is achieved so that you could form portions the size of golf balls with your hands. If the mix seems too dry to bind, then add a few drops of water. These delicious and filling little snacks can be kept in an airtight container in the refrigerator for weeks. Be careful not to eat too many as they are addictive.

Chapter 9: Social Events

Whether you socialize by choice or because you have a job that makes it a requirement, social events can really sabotage your healthy eating regime. For the healthy eater, it is not necessary to become a recluse, provided that you take a few simple precautions and as always remain mindful of what you eat and drink. Alcohol is always a problem when you are looking out for your health because it is high in sugar and, therefore, piles on the calories with practically no nutritional return. It also lowers your awareness of the food that you are taking in. I am not, however, going to promote teetotalism. When it comes to alcohol, beer, wine, and spirits are almost equally high in calories. Dry white wine tends to have slightly fewer calories and is the beverage I normally opt for when at business functions.

I try to take very small sips and drink slowly. I also have another trick that has served me well for years. I turn my white wine into a spritzer by adding sparkling water or soda. Often, at a function, I find that people will either insist that I drink or constantly top up my drink when it is only half empty. By topping up my wine with sparkling water, I am able to dramatically reduce the amount of wine that I consume without becoming a killjoy.

When sitting down to a meal that includes wine, I ask for a jug of water. In Europe, you will seldom go to a restaurant where water is not brought to the table automatically. After a glass of wine, I top up my glass with water that I also sip slowly. This naturally halves the amount of wine I consume while also making me feel full quicker.

Of course, food is the other big issue as your host or the restaurant you are visiting may not have the same attitude toward remaining healthy as you do. I believe that my decision to eat healthy food should not be imposed on others, and I would not like to be seen as one of those difficult people that need to have special meals provided for them. This is a guaranteed way to lose friends and reduce your social life, and that in itself is not conducive to a healthy lifestyle.

Here are a few tips to stay healthy while still having a social life.

Eat before you go out. If you have a light healthy meal before you go, you are much less likely to be tempted by those delicious but not-so-healthy offerings that are bound to be placed before you.

If you are serving yourself, dish up loads of salads and vegetables, and go easy on the food you are not sure about. Most social events will have salads, so use that to your advantage. If one doesn't have a salad, try finding the next, healthiest thing that you can find.

As always, eat slowly, and think about what you are eating. Remember to put your cutlery down between mouthfuls.

Drink lots of water, both to fill you up and to slow down your eating speed.

Unless the desert is something like a fruit salad, you may be better off opting for a piece of cheese rather that some very sweet dish.

Plan in advance about what you want to eat and try to find something on the menu that is compatible with your plan. You don't have to be too exact, but if you decide in advance that you are going to order something with ten percent protein, twenty percent starch, and the rest in vegetable, it should help guide you in what to order.

In many restaurants today, it seems almost obligatory to accompany any meal with a mound of French fries. Ask if you can have a salad or some vegetables instead. I find that restaurants will normally have some alternatives, and they have more frequently been beginning to cater toward clients who would like healthier options.

Try to chew every mouthful ten times, as this will slow down your eating rate and make your food easier to digest.

Don't be ashamed to leave some food on your plate. Remember that you are only eating until eighty percent full, and you should always be asking yourself, "Do I really want this?"

Engage people in conversation. It is harder to eat while you are talking, and it takes your mind away from feelings of hunger.

At stand up occasions, don't linger near the food table. Instead, wander throughout the room and try to start up a conversation with someone. Or, you can always find someplace where you can sit down and stay there instead of going to the food.

Try keeping one hand in your pocket and the other hand holding your glass. This will make it a little bit more difficult to reach for something off that passing tray of hors d'eurves. If nothing else, it will give you a second or two of extra time to reflect when that tray does come past. Olives or nuts are often healthy options when you feel you need something to nibble on.

If you absolutely cannot get away with doing these things, make the day of the social event your cheat day. That way, you won't feel so bad about the food you end up eating and can relax more. You shouldn't restrict yourself simply because you don't want to stray from your diet. Try to make this your cheat day and you'll notice that you are actually much happier and having more fun with the event.

Keep in mind that the very next day, you'll be back to your healthy eating. You don't need to panic as much if you know that you will definitely be eating healthy the next day. Plus, you can easily go and work out after the event if it's earlier in the day. Then, you'll be able to know that you did the best you could and still had fun at the event.

Finally, remember what we said about not beating yourself up and just carrying on the next day as though that bump in the road during the previous evening's dinner never happened.

Social events might seem like the end of your healthy eating sometimes. They don't have to be the worst thing in the world, however. They should be a fun time where you meet new people and maybe make some connections that will help further something you've been meaning to do. If you have a specific goal in mind for this social event, it might help keep your mind off of the food you're eating. Whatever happens, happens, so don't let yourself be upset over deciding to eat the dessert. It's always good to have one night of fun.

Chapter 10: The Importance Of Water

It might seem strange to be reading about water in a book on the subject of healthy eating, but water is one of the most neglected parts of our diet. Our bodies are made up of sixty percent water. Therefore, it very nearly makes up two-thirds of who we are. It also influences every single body process. With figures like that it suddenly makes more sense that we take a look at water intake and how it leads to healthier living.

Our bodies are constantly losing fluids. We do this through urination, through our skin when we perspire, and through respiration when we breathe. All of this fluid needs to be constantly replaced; otherwise, we become dehydrated. When we dehydrate, our bodies immediately start to function less efficiently. We need to balance fluid input with fluid output constantly, especially if we are living in or visiting warmer climates, exercising, or as we become older.

Our brain tells our kidneys how much fluid to release and how much to retain. The less we put in, the more the kidneys will retain fluid that contains impurities rather than allowing us to dehydrate. By drinking regularly, we ensure a constant through flow of clean fluids that aids just about every bodily function and improves not only our health, but also our overall sense of well-being. If you are feeling lethargic, try drinking a couple of glasses of chilled water with a slice of lemon or a sprig of mint, and see how quickly it picks you up. Dehydration, on the other hand, can actually cause the brain to shrink and reduce thought processes.

A great way to start drinking more water is simply by working out more often. If you don't work out consistently, you might notice that you just don't feel all that thirsty. Working out has the opposite effect. If you have a consistent workout routine, you'll notice that you are thirsty a lot more often. It might not be noticeable at first, but when you do notice it, you'll probably start drinking the recommended eight glasses a day.

We should not always wait until we are thirsty in order to have a drink. Older people are particularly prone to underestimating their own fluid intake, but all of us trying to maintain a healthy lifestyle should treat fluid intake as a form of purification for our systems. We have already discussed how drinking can help act as an appetite suppressant by filling us with a zero carbohydrate liquid, but below are few of the other health benefits to be had by drinking water.

Water keeps the skin looking its best. It not only hydrates the skin, but also flushes away impurities that may lead to skin problems, such as acne.

Bowl function is crucial to overall health, and water is great for maintaining healthy functioning bowels, especially when combined with the high fiber from the extra vegetables and fruit you are now eating.

When playing sports and exercising, our muscles perform better if they are properly hydrated. Hard exercise can build up lactic acid in the muscle fibers, and water improves the speed at which this acid is removed.

Water increases both energy and concentration levels.

The cartilage that surrounds our joints and our spinal columns is composed largely of water, and by keeping it fully lubricated, we improve our flexibility.

Tests have shown that high water intake may lead to a reduction in the risks of certain types of cancer and coronary disease.

Not all our fluid intake needs to come from drinking water. Eating fruit and vegetables increases our fluid intake, and so does drinking other liquids that we may prefer from time to time, such as tea or coffee (sorry, this does not include alcohol or sweet fizzy drinks). Remember that coffee is a diuretic, and as such, you may be losing more fluid than you take in. Try to keep your urine looking clear at all times. This is a good indicator that you are getting sufficient fluids. If your urine is clear or nearly clear when you go to the toilet first thing in the morning, then your fluid intake is brilliant, but don't drink so much late at night that you are forced to get up and go to the toilet during the night. Cool weather does not mean you will not be losing fluid. You may be perspiring less, but you will still be losing fluids through respiration.

Upping your water intake may take a bit of discipline at first. We have become accustomed to drinking only when we become thirsty as opposed to taking in fluid constantly throughout the day. Try having a water bottle on your desk, in your car, and with you when you perform sports. Also, take a glass of water every time you eat or have a snack. As with mindful eating, mindful drinking will help make you become more aware of what you consume, such that it eventually becomes a habit—one that is fundamental to good health.

Tea And Coffee

Both tea and coffee have been mainstay beverages for many people. Both beverages, but more so with coffee, received their share of bad press over the years in terms of their health benefits. People who consume these two drinks will be pleased to hear that in the 2015 edition of the Dietary Guidelines for Americans, caffeine was mentioned for the first time, and it was stated that drinking up to five cups of coffee per day was found to have no detrimental effects.

Both tea and coffee have certain health benefits, but they differ in what these benefits are.

Coffee

It improves short-term recall and may delay or prevent the onset of Alzheimer's disease.

It helps protect the liver from cirrhosis and liver cancer.

In men over the age of forty, it may help reduce the risk of gout.

It helps prevent the onset of Type II diabetes.

Tea

Tea is derived from the leaves of Camellia sinensis and is filled with anti-oxidants, which give it cancer-fighting properties.

Tea also has high levels of fluoride, which is good for the teeth.

Tea drinkers have shown reduced rates of heart attack, and tea may help prevent Type I diabetes.

People who drink four or more cups per day show lower levels of stress hormone.

In both cases, the beverage should be taken without milk or sugar as this reduces the benefits. Adding a slice of lemon to tea is desirable. Both of these drinks will help augment the amount of fluid you are consuming, but be aware that too much caffeine can have adverse effects, including anxiety, heart palpitations, and insomnia.

Nicholas Bjorn

Chapter 11: Healthy Eating And Children

Introducing your children to a healthy diet and getting them to stick to it is a challenging battle to enter into. Children are often more exposed to unhealthy foods than we are as adults. What is more is that there is an aggressive advertising campaign that targets children, who may spend much more of their lives watching television than adults do. Because they usually consume sugar and additive-filled drinks and sweet foods, they frequently have a more pronounced addiction to those than we may have.

Like us, kids need to be eating more whole foods and less processed foods, but they may not see the advantages of healthy eating habits in quite the same way as we do. They imagine themselves to be indestructible and have trouble realizing the long-term effects of what they eat.

On a more positive front, if we can get our kids hooked on healthy eating and help them move away from those tempting but unhealthy options at an early age, then we have a very good chance of setting them on the road to lifelong healthy living. Most experts agree that forcing them to go the healthy route is likely to be self-defeating in the long term. Instead, our kids should be encouraged.

Although we are pitted against a formidable enemy in this regard, we do have a few tricks at our disposal that may help us win this fight.

A great way to do this is to start them eating these healthy foods when they are very little, before they get exposed to the unhealthier foods. Making sure they have a wide variety of foods that are healthy when they are that age will almost guarantee that they will find one they like. They might even realize they like a lot of those foods, which will make it easier for you to cook for dinner. The younger that they are when you start them eating healthy, the more likely they'll eat that way throughout their life.

Family meals taken together at a regular time can have very positive effects. Children actually appreciate having a routine, and it helps develop their appetites when they know that they will be sitting down to a meal at a certain time. It also exposes them to other members of the family who are happily eating healthy food, which is great because children try to imitate adults.

Home cooking should become a base from which all healthy eating starts, and children will hopefully learn to appreciate food more if they are exposed to the love and effort that goes into it, as well as the wonderful aromas that fill the house whilst the food cooks. Try making simple meals so that the child can actually partake in the cooking and make a fuss of the results when they do. As they get older, they may be given one or two meals per week that they prepare alone.

When shopping, get the child interested in the choices that you make, and from the earliest age possible, let them begin to read the nutrition charts and learn to make informed decisions about which foods are good and which are not. Make sure that there are always some nutritious and healthy snacks for moments in the day when they need a little something between meals. When they are eating, restrict the quantity they are served, and don't force them to eat every item on their plates.

Total bans of sweets, ice cream, and other less healthy food may bring about resentment that could backfire at a later stage when children are old enough to be making food decisions on their own. Instead, give occasional treats, but also discuss with them what the healthy options are and what the results will be for those who abuse their bodies by flooding them with sugar, fat, and salt. Another great idea is to find alternative sweets that taste just as good as the sugary sweets they want. Some end up realizing that they want those more than the sugary ones.

Snacks should be healthy as much as possible. Instead of cookies, try giving them their favorite fruit or vegetable. If they eat healthy during their snack times, they might want to eat those foods during meal times as well. If you are able to, try buying organic foods. This way, you'll know what your child is eating and know that those foods don't have a lot of the preservatives that other foods have. Anything you can do to make your child's transition into eating healthy easier is something you should try. Of course, eating organic isn't something everyone can do, whether it be because of money or other reasons, but if you can, you should definitely try it out.

Sometimes, through no fault of your own, small children can be picky eaters, which is always a difficult problem to overcome and can lead to a lifetime of unbalanced and unhealthy eating habits. Below are a few methods that may be useful to try when you first start introducing your child to new foods.

Pick your time. Don't introduce anything new when the child is tired and likely to get difficult. Instead, offer the new ingredient when they have some energy and are both happy and hungry. Don't be too ambitious and try offering several new items at once. Let them discover the new items one at a time and become used to them before letting them broaden their horizons and move to the next food adventure.

Always try to make food fun. Turn the new food into a bit of an adventure, and make up some story to go with it if you think that will help. How many little boys were conned into eating tinned spinach because it gave Popeye the Sailor Man big muscles? By combining the new food with some more familiar favorites, you are less likely to meet with resistance.

Eat the food yourself. Kids love to copy their elders, and if they see you enjoying a dish, it won't be long before they want to give it a go. This is particularly true if they have been involved in the purchasing and preparing of the meal, and they feel they have a stake in the whole operation.

With smaller kids, disguising food can have wonderful results. Try making tomato soup and then putting a face on it with some blobs of cream. Get the child to make a picture using various vegetables to form trees and other images then get them to eat their picture. Making faces and pictures with food that is healthy soon gets young minds off the actual eating.

Fizzy drinks have an even worse effect on children than it does on adults as the ration of their body to the sugar content in these drinks is so much less. Tests have revealed that children who have four fizzy sodas per day are at a much higher risk of suffering from depression.

Don't assume that the meals that the school canteens are giving your child are as healthy as you would like them to be. Many large food companies have the contracts to supply canteens, and much of the food they provide is produced on an industrial scale with corresponding large quantities of sugar, salt, and preservatives. If you are unsure what the menus contain, then check, and if you are not satisfied, send your child his or her own lunch box with food that has more nutritious ingredients. Below are some easy options that you can prepare easily and which your child will enjoy. You may be surprised at just how much his or her concentration level increases when eating the right kinds of food.

Pita Bread Satchel:

Take pita bread, then cut it in half and stuff it with a mix of shredded chicken, chopped lettuce, and raisins coated with Greek yoghurt. This is a great way to use leftover chicken, and you can swap the raisins for halved grapes or diced apple.

Whole Wheat Bagel:

These guys are so useful for those instances when you are running out of time. Just slice your whole wheat bagel in half and spread peanut butter and a thin layer of honey.

Cinnamon Apple Chips:

Here is a great littler snack that keeps the kids away from potato crisps.

Thinly slice four crispy apples, mix enough granulated sugar and cinnamon to coat one side of your apple slices when they are spread out on a baking tray in a single layer. Bake for one hour in an oven that has been pre heated to 100 degrees C, and slowly bake for one hour. After one hour, turn them over and bake for a further hour, then turn off the oven but leave the apples inside. When the oven is cooled, the apple chips should be crisp and crunchy. If they are not, you may need to bake them for a further half hour. When they are cool, they will keep in an airtight container for a week.

Fruit And Yoghurt Ice Popsicles:

Tub of Greek yoghurt

Any mixed berries

Honey

Put the yoghurt and the berries in a blender, add a small amount of honey, and whiz everything together. Taste it for sweetness, and then, when you are happy with the flavor, spoon the mix into popsicle molds or small paper cups with a stick in the middle and pop them in the freezer for five hours. There are unlimited variations to this recipe. You could try adding chopped nuts or using vanilla flavored yoghurt. Whatever method you choose, your kids are bound to love it.

Chapter 12: Exercise

Whilst this is not a book on exercise, the importance of physical activity in terms of our overall health cannot be ignored, so I am going to give some brief pointers as to why we should exercise and the advantages it brings. I will also provide a few easy exercise options for those who don't want to rush off and invest in a gym membership or embark on a course of intense cardiovascular training routines. I am not decrying those options; it is just that this is not a book on that subject, and there is plenty of material available for those who wish to go down that road in greater depth. Certainly, when it comes to the subject of a healthy lifestyle, there is no question that a huge overlap exists between what we eat and how much we exercise.

Thirty minutes of light exercise a day has numerous health benefits, which we will look at shortly. A quick word of warning though for those who may not have exercised for a long time or who are suffering from a heart condition or other medical problem. It is always a good idea to consult your doctor before embarking on an exercise regime. If nothing else, it will give you peace of mind, and your medical practitioner will probably be able to suggest to what extreme you can safely push yourself.

Another very important factor when considering exercise it that it is no substitute for eating a well-balanced and controlled whole food diet. If you live in any modern city you will see people out there pounding the streets or pumping out hundreds of sit ups, imagining that they can work their bodies into one of those sculpted models they may have seen on television adverts for protein powder. To reduce weight by exercise alone requires a huge amount of time and effort. To put this into perspective, take jogging as an example. The average person jogging for one hour burns off three hundred calories. The average small chocolate bar contains two hundred and fifty calories. A can of coke (330ml) has one hundred and forty calories, and a similarly sized can of beer contains around one hundred calories. It does not take too long to work out that it would be very easy to regain all the calories lost in one hour, and a few extra to boot, with just a drink and so-called snack bar. So often, you see these poor misguided people sweating away and getting nowhere in terms of losing weight, simply because they lack an understanding of how their bodies work.

Please don't misunderstand me here. I am all in favor of exercise, but moderate exercise in combination with a healthy diet far outweighs heavy exercise and an unhealthy diet every time. What is more, many of those people slogging away at their fitness routine are probably increasing their appetites and taking on more calories than they otherwise might have done.

Here are some of the advantages of moderate exercise and why you should consider it in conjunction with the healthy eating habits you have learned in this book.

Exercise Advantages

You will burn more calories if you exercise, and provided you don't replace those with increased eating, you will lose weight faster. It is not necessary to engage yourself in aerobic classes or join a running club to increase the amount of exercise you do on a daily basis. Just taking the stairs as opposed to the elevator or getting off your bus one stop further from your destination than you usually do can add to the amount you exercise you do over the course of a week. A half hour's walk three or four times a week can soon turn into a pleasure rather than a chore, and you can increase the speed as you get fitter.

Exercise boosts blood HDL or good cholesterol. The increase in metabolic rate when exercise is done on a regular basis dramatically reduces the risk of cardiac disease.

It might seem counterintuitive, but regular exercise increases your overall energy levels. The extra oxygen flowing through your system strengthens muscle tissues, boosts brain activity, and improves your heart rate.

Extra exercise will also improve the quality of your sleep. Sleep deprivation is a growing problem for many people, and it carries with it a raft of health problems in itself. Exercise is a great way to sleep better, but try not to do your exercise in the last hour before you sleep, given that the higher metabolic rate that the exercise induces may stop you going to sleep straight away.

Exercise does wonders for our minds. It is a great way to alleviate depression and get rid of those feelings of lethargy that a more sedentary lifestyle can induce. Moderate exercise increases the amount of endorphins going to our brains. These are a group of hormones secreted within the nervous system that are particularly important when it comes to mood enhancement.

Being fitter improves our overall sense of self-esteem. The importance of self-esteem should never be underestimated because when we feel good about ourselves and the way we look, it gives us the inspiration and confidence to do even more to maintain our health.

Despite the views you may have to the contrary, possibly as a result of uninspiring of even humiliating childhood physical exercise lessons, sport can be fun. It is a wonderful means by which to be exposed to nature or to interact with both family and friends.

Finally, exercise even has benefits in terms of our sex lives. It increases sex drive and can reduce the incidence of erectile dysfunction in men. Men might notice that they tend to have a higher sex drive after they've worked out, which is attributed to the exercise itself. It gets your blood pumping and your muscles working. There will also be a release of endorphins that will add to the sex drive.

Gone are the days where the only way to exercise meant going to expensive gyms or having to purchase specialist clothing that may not have looked flattering on anyone that was not already super fit. There are now a number of internet workout routines that one can perform in the privacy of one's own bedroom. If that is not your cup of tea, why not just do a bit more walking, either in your own neighborhood or some of the many walking trails that are being rolled out around the country and in many cities. A walk of two miles will burn off almost exactly the same amount of calories as a jog of two miles, though with considerable less shock to the joints. Whatever routine you opt for, make sure it is pleasurable and remember that it is only an enhancement of your healthy eating regime and is not intended to replace it.

At Home Exercises

Here are a few at home exercises that you'll be able to do away from prying eyes. Not everyone is comfortable with going straight to a gym to do all of these things, so starting with some at home exercises might be exactly what you need.

For one, you need to keep in mind that cardio is a great way to help you burn fat. Generally, cardio tends to be a full-body workout. When you go for a jog, you are using your legs, arms, and core to keep at a steady pace. For every hour you jog, you burn around 300 calories. While jogging might not be for everyone, it is a very effective exercise and should be kept in the back of your mind. Another great exercise is using a jump rope. This is definitely a cardio workout and will get your whole body moving. Not only is it a great fat-burning workout, but it can also improve your agility and help you if you want to be on a sports team or are on a sports team. Jumping rope for half an hour (which isn't recommended) can burn up to 480 calories. It can also help your breathing efficiency, since you eventually start to breathe a lot heavier when you jump rope for an extended period of time.

If you want to specifically target your belly fat, then try what's called the superman exercise. With this exercise, you lay on the ground, your stomach touching the ground. Make sure your arms are straight in front of you, stretched as far as they can go. Then, lift your legs and chest off the ground, your arms going up with your chest. Try to hold this position for thirty seconds, keeping your chest and legs as high up as they can go. Make sure your glutes are tightened along with your abs to ensure that you won't pull your lower back. Then, release and bring everything back to the ground. It not only works your core muscles, but also your thighs and lower back. Doing this exercise a few times throughout your workout would make it effective.

Here's another great cardio exercise, one that will be plenty of fun to do. It is called the jump squat exercise. Your whole body gets worked, but it's a great for toning your thighs as well. It's pretty easy to guess what this exercise likely entails. All you need to do is stand straight with your hands behind your head. Then, bend your legs and try to get into a perfect squat position. As you start to go back up, go into a jump instead. Right as you land, already start going back into a squat. This exercise is pretty intense and it makes for a great fat-burning exercise. Doing this in your routine every day will make a huge difference in your body shape.

Maybe push-ups aren't your cup of tea. They can be rather monotonous and some people just don't see them as all that interesting. What if there was a way to spice up your push-ups and make them more interesting? Try doing the push-up and knee kick exercise and it might be your new favorite way to do a push-up. For this, you need to start in a push-up position. Then, do a single push-up. Take your right leg and bend it to touch your right elbow. Bring it back and do the same with your left leg. Then, do another push-up. This exercise is especially effective on your upper arms and will help you lose that fat. This can be a hard place to lose fat, so it's nice to have this exercise to work that area.

Another great variation of push-up is the lunge to push-up. This works quite a few parts of your body, from your chest and shoulders to your butt and legs, plus your abs and arms. It makes this a full body workout that you will grow to love. To start, stand with your feet hip width apart and your hands on your hips. From there, you need to put your right foot forward and go down into a lunge. Instead of coming back up, lean over your right knee and put your hands on the ground on either side. Step your right foot back, bringing yourself into a push-up position. Then, do a push-up. Bring your right foot forward again and bring yourself back into a lunge position. Finally, come back up to your starting position, with your hands on your hips. You can then switch and do your left leg. If you can, try to do this at least ten times. That means going down into the lunge on both sides and doing two push-ups altogether for it to count as one. These are really wonderful push-ups to try out.

If you want to focus a little more on your glutes and core, try the glute bridge. This exercise specifically targets these two areas and also helps tone your calves, hamstrings, flexors, and lower back. For this exercise, lay down on your back and bend your knees up, your feet flat on the floor. Raise your hips up and form a straight line from your knees to your chest. From there, lift your right leg up, keeping it bent, and try to get as close to your chest as possible. Hold this for a few seconds before lowering your leg back down. Then, repeat with your left leg. You can then lower your hips back down to the ground. This is also an effective way to relieve back pain and can take the place of any of the yoga back pain relief poses. You can repeat this as many times as you desire, so have fun with it!

The alternating lunge is another great idea for an exercise. This is probably a familiar one to you, but it is very effective. Lunges, in general, are used in a lot of calisthenics routines since they are such a good way to burn calories and lose weight. It not only focuses on the legs, but also the abdomen, lower back, and core. To do this exercise, start standing up straight with your hands on your hips. This will give you a nice balance when you go into the lunge. Move your right leg forward and bend your body down. Make sure your right leg stays perpendicular when you go down into the lunge. Come back up and stand straight again. Then, put your left leg forward and go down into a lunge on that side. For the best results repeat this as many times as you can in one minute, making sure to go down fully with your lunges.

Here's another great exercise for your legs and your core. It's called the W Leg Lifts exercise. For this to be the most effective, you need to make sure to tighten your core as you swing your legs up. Otherwise, you won't be getting much out of this exercise and you're more likely to hurt yourself. To start, lay on your back with your hands at your sides. Take a moment to just relax. Then, making sure your legs are together, tighten your core and raise your legs up. If you can, try to make sure they are directly above you, making an L shape with your body. Bring them back down about halfway and then go back up. Do this as many times as you can in thirty seconds. You'll definitely feel the burn as you start doing this. When you get stronger, you can up the time to a minute, as this will give your body an extra push.

Do you want an exercise that will really work all of your abdominal muscles? Try the rotating T extension. This exercise really does work every single one of your abdominal muscles, making it a great exercise for strengthening your core to its full potential. With this, you need to start in the push-up position, but with your arms straight up. Then, shift your weight from both of your arms to just your left. Bring your body so that your right arm goes straight up and you are facing that arm. This makes a T shape with your body. Your right foot should be on top of your left as well. Then, slowly come back down into the push-up position and do the same with your left side. Try to do this as many times as possible in one minute. If you can't keep your balance, then just try to go through it slowly and have your body figure out exactly what it needs to do. Throughout the exercise, make sure to keep your core tightened. That is the best way to get the abs that you want from doing this exercise.

Another great arm exercise is the reverse dip. You will need something like a stable chair or bench in order to do this exercise properly. For this, sit in front of the bench and put your hands on the top of it. Using your arms, push up so you are in a sitting position, but without anything underneath your butt. Slowly lower yourself down, bending your arms to around a ninety degree angle. Be sure to not let your butt touch the ground as you go down as that will end up negating the work you had just done. Then, push yourself back up to your starting position. Try to do this as many times as possible in a minute. It's a great workout for your arms and your legs. There is a squatting part to this exercise that will really work your lower body.

Of course, it doesn't matter how much exercise you do. If you want to truly be fit and healthy, you also need to eat healthy. Working out and eating like crap won't be beneficial. Eating really well and not working out won't be beneficial. Mixing the two together, however, will yield results that you will be very happy about. It is always best when you do a mix of both rather than doing one over the other.

Below, there is a sample meal plan for you to try out. This plan gives you all the nutrition you need to not only have a good and healthy body, but also give you the energy that you need to do all the exercises you have planned. If you find that you need to substitute anything due to a food allergy, try to find a food that has similar nutrients and will be just as beneficial.

5-Day Sample Meal Plan

Day 1

Breakfast: Grapefruit, Eggs

Morning Snack: Whole Grain Bagel and Peanut Butter

Lunch: Turkey Rolls with Tomatoes and Cheese

Afternoon Snack: Tuna (in water) and Cottage Cheese

Dinner: Stir Fry Vegetables, Shrimp, Ginger Root, and Mixed Green Salad in Balsamic Vinegar

Late Night Snack: Walnut Halves

Day 2

Breakfast: 2 Large Whole Eggs, Cooked Oatmeal, and Extra Lean Bacon

Morning Snack: Whole Bread and Peanut Butter

Lunch: Chicken Breasts and Mixed Green Salad in Balsamic Vinegar

Afternoon Snack: Reduced Fat Greek Yogurt, Handful of Almonds

Dinner: Mixed Frozen Vegetables, Salmon and Mixed Greens in Balsamic Vinegar

Late Night Snack: Cottage Cheese

Day 3

Breakfast: 2 Large Whole Eggs, Cottage Cheese, 1 Whole Grain Waffle, and 2 Tbsp. Fat-Free Whipped Cream

Morning Snack: 1 Apple and Peanut Butter

Lunch: Tuna (In Water) and Mixed Greens in Balsamic Vinegar

Afternoon Snack: 2 Slices Low Fat Ham, Low Fat American Cheese and ¼ Avocado

Dinner: Chopped Broccoli, Chicken Breasts and Mixed Greens in Balsamic Vinegar

Late Night Snack: Cottage Cheese

Day 4

Breakfast: Grapefruit and Eggs

Morning Snack: Turkey Breasts, Cottage Cheese, and Walnut Halves

Lunch: Tuna (in water) and Mixed Greens in Balsamic Vinegar

Afternoon Snack: Light Mozzarella String Cheese

Dinner: Lean Ground Turkey, Fat Free Cheddar Cheese, Fat Free Sour Cream, Shredded Iceberg Lettuce, Salsa, and Diced Medium Tomato

Late Night Snack: Walnut Halves

Day 5

Breakfast: Lean Cereal, Low Fat Milk, and Whole Eggs (fried or scrambled in olive oil)

Morning Snack: Boiled Soybeans and Light Mozzarella String Cheese

Lunch: Cottage Cheese

Afternoon Snack: Shrimp With Spicy Cocktail Sauce

Dinner: Chili Con Carne And Mixed Greens in Balsamic Vinegar

Late Night Snack: Medium Celery Stalks and Peanut Butter

Conclusion

Thank you again for purchasing this book!

I hope this book was able to help you understand what nutrition is about and how it can benefit your health and your life.

The next step is to apply what you have just read in this book by making sure that the next time you go to the grocery store, you buy the right kinds of foods. This means checking nutritional labels to select the healthiest foods possible.

If you've enjoyed this book, then I'd like to ask you for a favor. Would you be kind enough to leave a review for this book on Amazon? It would be greatly appreciated!

Thank you so much and good luck!

Nicholas Bjorn

CPSIA information can be obtained
at www.ICGtesting.com
Printed in the USA
BVOW06s0421230117
474158BV00021B/78/P

9 781519 485496